Fitness & Wellness

Third Edition

Werner W. K. Hoeger

Boise State University

Sharon A. Hoeger

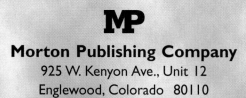

Morton Publishing Company

925 W. Kenyon Ave., Unit 12
Englewood, Colorado 80110

Acknowledgments

The authors wish to thank Dr. Ross Vaughn for writing the new section on Biomechanics and Dr. James Nicholson for providing materials for the section on Motivation and Behavior Modification. Special gratitude to Charles Scheer, Erin C. Caskey, David T. Aschenbrener, Matt McKain, and Welsh Studios for their help with the photography for this new edition.

Morton Publishing Company would like to thank you, our second edition users, for the many ideas and suggestions you provided for this new third edition. We appreciate your continued support and look forward to serving you again in the future.

Printed in the United States of America

10   9   8   7   6   5   4   3   2

ISBN: 0-89582-319-5

Preface

More than ever before Americans realize that good health is largely self-controlled and that premature illness and mortality can be prevented through adequate fitness and positive lifestyle habits.

The current American way of life, unfortunately, does not provide the human body with sufficient physical activity to maintain adequate health. Furthermore, many present lifestyle patterns are such a serious threat to our health that they actually increase the deterioration rate of the human body and often lead to premature illness and mortality.

Several major scientific research studies indicate that people who lead an active and healthy lifestyle live longer and enjoy a better quality of life. As a result, the importance of sound fitness and wellness programs has assumed an entirely new dimension. From an initial fitness fad in the early 1970s, healthy lifestyle programs have become a trend that is now very much a part of the American way of life.

Nevertheless, while people in the United States are firm believers in the benefits of exercise and positive lifestyle habits as a means to promote better health, most do not reap these benefits because they do not know how to implement a sound fitness and wellness program that will yield the desired results. Therefore, the information presented in this book has been written with this purpose in mind: to provide you with the necessary guidelines to implement a lifetime exercise and healthy lifestyle program so you can make a constant and deliberate effort to stay healthy and realize your highest potential for well-being.

ENHANCED FEATURES OF THE THIRD EDITION

The chapters in the **third edition** of *Fitness & Wellness* have been revised and updated to include new information reported in the literature and at professional health, physical education, and sportsmedicine meetings. A questionnaire was given to almost all users of the second edition to evaluate the book. The recommendations made proved extremely valuable in the preparation of this new edition. While it was difficult to include all of the suggestions, the great majority were addressed. The most significant changes of the third edition are:

❖ The book now contains eight chapters instead of seven. Because of the extensiveness of the information on nutrition and weight management, this chapter is divided into two separate chapters. This change allows for greater discussion of these topics.

❖ Chapter 1 has been extensively revised and now includes a much broader discussion on wellness and the dimensions of wellness, the U.S. Health Objectives for the Year 2000 (objectives that emphasize the need for health promotion and disease prevention, personal responsibility, and health benefits for all people in the United States), an introduction to the motor skill-related components of fitness, essential information on motivation and behavior modification to help students implement a lifetime wellness program, an update on the association between fitness and mortality, the relevance of initiating and adhering to a fitness/wellness program during youth, and the effects of a healthy lifestyle on quality of life and longevity.

❖ A new abdominal crunch test has been included in Chapter 2. This test replaces the previously used abdominal curl-up test.

❖ The cardiorespiratory endurance and muscular strength exercise prescriptions in Chapter 3 have been revised to conform with the 1995

Guidelines for Exercise Testing and Prescription by the American College of Sports Medicine (ACSM). This chapter now also contains an introduction to biomechanical principles related to cardiorespiratory activities and muscular strength and endurance activities.

❖ A new exercise modality: "Aero-belt Exercise" was added to Chapter 4. The significance of motor-skill related fitness and an analysis of the contributions of selected activities to skill-fitness components were also included.

❖ New information and revisions were made to the nutrition chapter, including extensive information on antioxidants, phytochemicals, new food labels, and daily values.

❖ The list of food items in Appendix E has been expanded to 479 food items. Most of the new additions to this list are commonly eaten fast-food items.

❖ A broader discussion of the terms obesity, overweight, recommended weight, and "tolerable" weight is included in the weight loss chapter. Such information helps students make an informed decision as to what constitutes a realistic target weight.

❖ Based on latest research reports, the importance of physical activity as a major factor, if not the most important one, in prevention of obesity and maintenance of recommended body weight has been enhanced in the weight management chapter.

❖ Major revisions have been made to the healthy lifestyle chapter (Chapter 7) to incorporate recent advances in this area, in particular as related to cardiovascular diseases and cancer. The section on tension and stress was also enhanced and the material on HIV and AIDS have been expanded.

❖ Information on exercise clothing; overtraining; guidelines for the prevention of consumer fraud; factors to consider when selecting a health/fitness club; issues related to the selection, purchase, and maintenance of exercise equipment; and reliable sources for health/fitness information have been included in Chapter 8.

❖ New color photography and outstanding new graphs have been added throughout the book.

SUPPLEMENTS

The following ancillaries are provided free of charge to all qualified *Fitness & Wellness* adopters:

❖ A **comprehensive computer software package**. This package includes a *Fitness Profile*, a *Personalized Cardiorespiratory Exercise Prescription*, a *Nutrient Analysis*, and a weekly and monthly *Exercise Log*. The fitness profile provides a pre- and post-test comparison, including percent change for each fitness item on the profile. This software package provides a more meaningful experience for all participants.

A new feature of the third edition is the *Nutrient Analysis Data Base Enhancer* software. This software allows course instructors to add food items to the already existing data base available with the book.

❖ A **video** containing a detailed explanation of many of the fitness assessment test items used in the book. Instructors can use this video to help familiarize themselves with the proper test protocols for each fitness test. This audio-visual aid contains the following test items: 1.5-Mile Run Test, Muscular Endurance Test, Modified Sit-and-Reach Test, Body Rotation Test, and Skinfold Thickness Test.

❖ The Physical Fitness and Wellness **Computerized Testbank** with the following options: (a) Over 800 multiple choice questions, (b) capability to add/or edit test questions, (c) previously generated tests can be recalled — creating new exam versions — because multiple-choice answers can be rotated with each new test generated, and (d) capability to generate tests using a LaserJet printer.

❖ Sixty-four color **overhead transparency acetates**, including some of the book's most important illustrations and tables to facilitate class instruction and help explain key fitness and wellness concepts.

❖ An **instructor's manual** to aid with implementation of your physical fitness and wellness course.

Contents

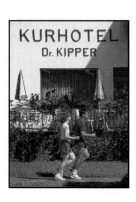
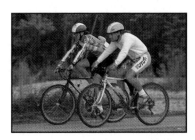
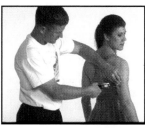

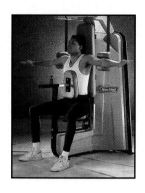
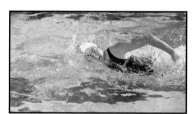
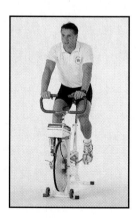

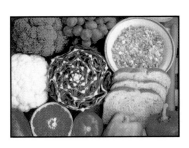

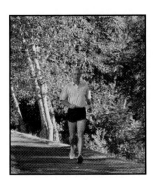

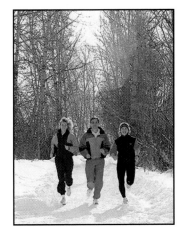

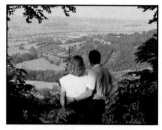

8 Relevant Questions and Answers to Fitness and Wellness   145

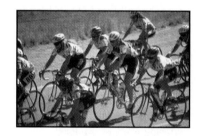

APPENDICES

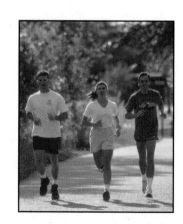

CHAPTER 1

The Importance of Physical Fitness and Wellness

There is no drug in current or prospective use that holds as much promise for sustained health as a lifetime program of physical exercise.[1]

KEY TERMS

Behavior modification

Chronic diseases

Epidemiology

Health-related fitness

Hypokinetic diseases

Locus of control

Motivation

Physical fitness

Skill-related fitness

Wellness

OBJECTIVES

❖ Understand the importance of physical fitness.

❖ Understand the wellness concept.

❖ Define physical fitness and list health-related and skill-related fitness components.

❖ Learn the benefits of a total fitness and wellness program.

❖ Learn motivation and behavior modification techniques to enhance compliance with a fitness and wellness program.

❖ Determine whether medical clearance is required for safe participation in exercise.

Most people go to college to learn how to make a living, but a fitness and wellness course will teach you how to live — how to truly live life to its fullest potential. Some people seem to think that success in life is measured by how much money they make. Making a good living will not help you unless you live a wellness lifestyle that will allow you to enjoy what you have.

Everyone would like to enjoy good health and wellness, but most people don't know how to reach this objective. Lifestyle is the most important factor affecting our personal well-being. Although some people live long because of genetic factors, the quality of life during middle age and the "golden years" is related more often to wise choices initiated during youth and continued throughout life.

During the last three decades the number of people participating in physical fitness programs has increased tremendously. The initial fitness fad in the early 1970s turned into a trend that has become part of the American way of life. The increase in the number of fitness participants is attributed primarily to scientific evidence linking increased physical activity and positive lifestyle habits to better health and improved quality of life.

Unfortunately, the current American way of life does not provide the human body with sufficient physical exercise to maintain adequate health. Furthermore, many lifestyle patterns are such a serious threat to our health that they actually increase the deterioration of the human body. In a few short years lack of wellness leads to a loss of vitality and gusto for life, as well as premature morbidity and mortality.

The "typical" American is not a good role model when cardiorespiratory fitness is concerned. Almost 60% of U.S. adults engage in little or no leisure-time physical activity. In 1994, only 37% of the adults in the United States exercised strenuously three or more days per week.[2] Even though people in the United States believe that a positive lifestyle has a great impact on health and longevity, most do not reap the benefits because they don't know how to implement a fitness and wellness program that will yield the desired results.

Patty Neavill is a typical example of someone who frequently tried to change her life around but was unable to do so because she did not know how to implement a sound exercise and weight control program. At age 24, Patty, a college sophomore, was discouraged with her weight, level of fitness, self-image, and quality of life in general. She had struggled with weight most of her life. Like thousands of other people, she had made many unsuccessful attempts to

lose weight. Patty put her fears aside and decided to enroll in a fitness course. As part of the course requirement, she took a battery of fitness tests at the beginning of the semester. Patty's cardiorespiratory fitness and strength ratings were poor, her flexibility classification was average, she weighed more than 200 pounds, and her percent body fat was 41.

Following the initial fitness assessment, Patty met with her course instructor, who prescribed an exercise and nutrition program like the one in this book. Patty fully committed to carry out the prescription. She walked or jogged five times a week, worked out with weights twice a week, and played volleyball or basketball two to four times each week. Her daily caloric intake was set in the range of 1,500 to 1,700 calories. She took care to meet the minimum required servings from the basic food groups each day, which contributed about 1,200 calories to her diet. The remainder of the calories came primarily from complex carbohydrates. At the end of the 16-week semester, Patty's cardiorespiratory fitness, strength, and flexibility ratings had all improved to the good category, she lost 50 pounds, and her percent body fat had dropped to 22.5!

A thank-you note from Patty to the course instructor at the end of the semester read:

> Thank you for making me a new person. I truly appreciate the time you spent with me. Without your kindness and motivation, I would have never made it. It's great to be fit and trim. I've never had this feeling before and I wish everyone could feel like this once in their life.
>
> > Thank you,
> > Your trim Patty!

Patty never had been taught the principles governing a sound weight loss program. Not only did she need this knowledge, but, like most Americans who never have experienced the process of becoming physically fit, she needed to be in a structured exercise setting to truly feel the joy of fitness.

Of even greater significance, Patty has maintained her aerobic and strength-training programs. A year after ending her calorie-restricted diet, her weight increased by 10 pounds, but her body fat decreased from 22.5% to 21.2%. As discussed in Chapter 6, the weight increase is related mostly to changes in lean tissue, lost during the weight-reduction phase. Despite only a slight drop in weight during the second year following the calorie-restricted diet, the 2-year follow-up revealed a further decrease in body fat, to 19.5%. Patty understands the new quality of life reaped through a sound fitness program.

LIFESTYLE, HEALTH, AND QUALITY OF LIFE

Many research findings have shown that physical inactivity and negative lifestyle habits pose a serious threat to health. Movement and physical activity are basic functions for which the human organism was created. Now, however, advances in modern technology have all but eliminated the need for physical activity in almost everyone's daily life.

Physical activity is no longer a natural part of our existence. Today we live in an automated society. Most of the activities that used to require strenuous physical exertion can be accomplished by machines with the simple pull of a handle or push of a button. For instance, if people need to go to a store that is only a couple of blocks away, most drive their automobiles and then spend a couple of minutes driving

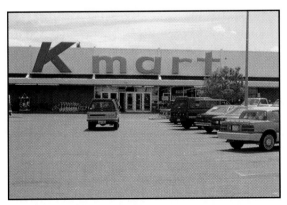

The epitome of physical inactivity: driving around a parking lot for several minutes in search of a parking spot 10 to 20 yards closer to the store's entrance.

around the parking lot to find a spot 10 yards closer to the store's entrance. The groceries do not even have to be carried out any more. They usually are taken out in a cart and placed in the vehicle by a youngster working at the store.

Similarly, during a visit to a multi-level shopping mall, nearly everyone chooses to ride the escalators instead of taking the stairs. Automobiles, elevators, escalators, telephones, intercoms, remote controls, electric garage door openers — all are modern-day commodities that minimize the amount of movement and effort required of the human body.

One of the most significant detrimental effects of modern-day technology has been an increase in *chronic conditions related to a lack of physical activity*. These include hypertension, heart disease, chronic low-back pain, and obesity, among others They sometimes are referred to as hypokinetic diseases. "Hypo" means low or little, and "kinetic" implies motion. Lack of adequate physical activity is a fact of modern life that most people can no longer avoid, but to enjoy contemporary commodities and still expect to live life to its fullest, a personalized lifetime exercise program must become a part of daily living.

With the developments in technology, three additional factors have changed our lives significantly and have had a negative effect on human health: nutrition, stress, and environment. Fatty foods, sweets, alcohol, tobacco, excessive stress, and environmental hazards such as wastes, noise, and air pollution have detrimental effects on people.

The most prominent causes of death in the United States today are lifestyle-related (see Figure 1.1). Current statistics indicate that approximately 66% of all deaths in the United States are caused by cardiovascular disease and cancer.[3] Nearly 80% of these deaths could be prevented by adhering to a healthy lifestyle. The third cause of death, chronic and obstructive pulmonary disease (COPD), is related largely to tobacco use. Accidents comprise the fourth leading cause of death. Even though not all accidents are preventable, many are. Fatal accidents

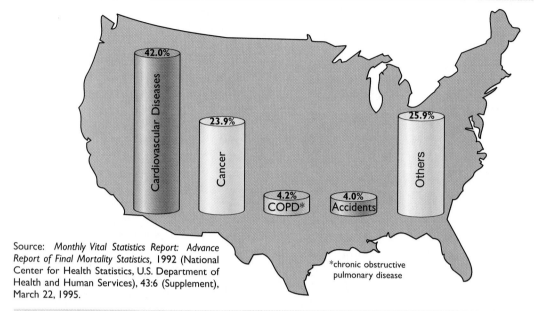

Source: *Monthly Vital Statistics Report: Advance Report of Final Mortality Statistics,* 1992 (National Center for Health Statistics, U.S. Department of Health and Human Services), 43:6 (Supplement), March 22, 1995.

*chronic obstructive pulmonary disease

FIGURE 1.1 ✿ Leading causes of death in the United States, 1992.

often are related to abusing drugs and not wearing seat belts.

As the incidence of chronic diseases — *illnesses that develop and last over a long time* — increased, it became obvious that prevention was the best medicine. Estimates indicate that more than half of disease is lifestyle-related, a fifth is attributed to the environment, and a tenth is influenced by the health care the individual receives. Only 16% is related to genetic factors.[4] Thus, the individual controls 84% of disease and quality of life. Further, according to estimates, 83% of deaths before age 65 are preventable. In essence, most Americans are threatened by the very lives they lead today.

Ideally, healthy lifestyle habits should be taught and reinforced in early youth. Unfortunately, many young people are in such poor physical condition that they will add to national health concerns in years to come. Surveys conducted during the past decade have raised public concern regarding the fitness level of American youth. As compared to the 1960s and 1970s, cardiorespiratory endurance and upper body

strength have decreased and body fat has increased. These findings suggest that current physical education programs are not promoting lifetime fitness and wellness adequately.

Although the incidence of cardiovascular disease has declined remarkably in the last two decades, concern over youth fitness has led Dr. Kenneth Cooper, Director of the Aerobics Research Institute in Dallas, Texas to state: "It's discouraging and I am afraid that as these kids grow up, we will see all the gains made against heart disease in the last twenty years wiped out in the next twenty years."[5] Even 5- and 6-year-old children already have coronary heart disease risk factors such as high blood pressure, excessive body fat, and low fitness.[6]

Because of the unhealthy lifestyles that many young adults lead, physically they may be middle-aged or older! Healthy choices made today influence health a decade or two later. Many physical education programs do not emphasize the necessary skills for our youth to maintain a high level of fitness and health throughout life. That is the intent of this book — to provide the skills and help to prepare you for a lifetime of physical fitness and wellness. A healthy lifestyle is self-controlled, and people need to be taught how to be responsible for their own health and fitness.

WELLNESS

After the initial fitness boom swept across the country in the 1970s, it became clear that improving physical fitness alone was not always enough to lower the risk for disease and ensure better health. For example, individuals who run 3 miles a day, lift weights regularly, participate in stretching exercises, and watch their body weight can be classified readily as having good or excellent fitness. If these same people, however, have high blood pressure, smoke, are under constant stress, consume too much alcohol, and eat too many fatty foods, they are at risk for cardiovascular disease and may not be aware of it. The characteristics that predict the development of a certain disease are called *risk factors*.

Good health is no longer viewed as simply the absence of illness. The notion of good health has evolved notably in the last few years and continues to change as scientists learn more about lifestyle factors that bring on illness and affect wellness. Once the idea took hold that fitness by itself would not always decrease the risk for disease and ensure better health, the wellness concept developed in the 1980s.

Wellness is defined as *the constant and deliberate effort to stay healthy and achieve the highest potential for well-being*. Wellness is an all-inclusive umbrella covering a variety of health-related factors. Wellness living requires the implementation of positive programs to change behavior and thereby improve health and quality of life, prolong life, and achieve total well-being.

To enjoy a wellness lifestyle, a person needs to practice behaviors that will lead to positive outcomes in five dimensions of wellness: physical, emotional, intellectual, social, and spiritual (Figure 1.2). These dimensions are interrelated;

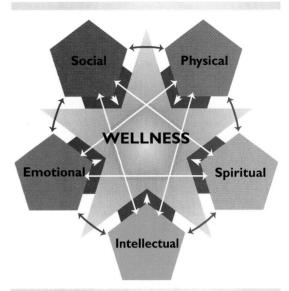

FIGURE 1.2 ❖ The dimensions of wellness.

one frequently affects the others. For example, a person who is emotionally "down" often has no desire to exercise, study, socialize with friends, or attend church.

In looking at the five dimensions of wellness, high-level wellness clearly goes beyond the absence of disease and optimal fitness. Wellness incorporates components such as fitness, proper nutrition, stress management, disease prevention, social support, self-worth, nurturance (sense of being needed), spirituality, smoking cessation, personal safety, substance control, regular physical examinations, health education, and environmental support.

For a wellness way of life, individuals not only must be physically fit and manifest no signs of disease but also must have no risk factors for disease (such as physical inactivity, hypertension, abnormal cholesterol levels, cigarette smoking, negative stress, faulty nutrition, careless sex). Even though an individual tested in a fitness center may demonstrate adequate or even excellent fitness, indulgence in unhealthy lifestyle behaviors still will increase the risk for chronic diseases and decrease the person's well-being. Additional information on wellness and how to implement a wellness program is discussed in Chapter 7.

Unhealthy behaviors are contributing to the staggering U.S. health care costs. Risk factors for disease carry a heavy price tag (see Table 1.1). About 1 trillion dollars were spent in health care costs alone in 1994. According to estimates,[7] 1% of Americans account for 30% of these costs. Half of the people use up about 97% of the health care dollars.

PHYSICAL FITNESS

The American Medical Association defines physical fitness as *the general capacity to adapt and respond favorably to physical effort*. This implies that individuals are physically fit when they can meet both the ordinary and the unusual demands of daily life safely and effectively without being overly fatigued and still have energy left for leisure and recreational activities. Physical fitness can be classified into health-related and motor-skill-related fitness.

TABLE 1.1 ✣ Average Annual Health Care Costs for Leading Disease Risk Factors

Risk Factor	Annual Cost
Smoking	$960
Obesity	$401
Excessive alcohol use	$389
High blood pressure	$373
High cholesterol	$370
Not using seat belts	$272

Source: *Journal of Occupational Medicine*, November 1991.

Health-Related Fitness

Health-related fitness *has four components* (see Figure 1.3) *cardiorespiratory endurance, muscular strength and endurance, muscular flexibility, and body composition*:

1. *Cardiorespiratory endurance*: the ability of the heart, lungs, and blood vessels to supply

Cardiorespiratory Endurance

Muscular Flexibility

Body Composition

Muscular Strength and Endurance

FIGURE 1.3 ✣ Health-related components of physical fitness.

oxygen to the cells to meet the demands of prolonged physical activity (also referred to as aerobic exercise).

2. *Muscular strength and endurance*: the ability of the muscles to generate force.

3. *Muscular flexibility*: the capacity of a joint to move freely through a full range of motion.

4. *Body composition*: the amount of lean body mass and adipose tissue (fat mass) in the human body.

Skill-Related Fitness

The motor skill-related components of fitness are important for successful motor performance in athletic events and in lifetime sports and activities such as basketball, racquetball, golf, hiking, soccer, and water skiing. Good skill-related fitness also enhances overall quality of life by helping people cope more effectively in emergency situations (see Chapter 4). The components of skill-related fitness are agility, balance, coordination, power, reaction time, and speed (see Figure 1.4):

1. *Agility*: the ability to change body position and direction quickly and efficiently. Agility is important in sports such as basketball, soccer, and racquetball, in which the participant must change direction rapidly and at the same time maintain proper body control.

2. *Balance*: the ability to maintain the body in equilibrium. Balance is vital in activities such as gymnastics, diving, ice skating, skiing, and even football and wrestling, in which the athlete attempts to upset the opponent's equilibrium.

3. *Coordination*: integration of the nervous system and the muscular system to produce correct, graceful, and harmonious body movements. This component is important in a wide variety of motor activities such as golf, baseball, karate, soccer, and racquetball, in which hand-eye or foot-eye movements, or both, must be integrated.

4. *Power*: the ability to produce maximum force in the shortest time. The two components of power are *speed* and *force* (strength). An effective combination of these two components allows a person to produce explosive movements such as in jumping, putting the shot, and spiking/throwing/hitting a ball.

5. *Reaction time*: the time required to initiate a response to a given stimulus. Good reaction time is important for starts in track and swimming, to react quickly when playing tennis at the net, and in sports such as ping pong, boxing, and karate.

6. *Speed*: the ability to propel the body or a part of the body rapidly from one point to another. Sprints in track, stealing a base in baseball, soccer, and basketball are examples of activities that require good speed for success.

In terms of preventive medicine, the main emphasis of fitness programs should be on the health-related components. Although skill-related fitness is crucial for success in sports and athletics, it also contributes to wellness. Improving skill-related fitness not only affords an individual more enjoyment and success in lifetime sports, but regular participation in skill-fitness activities also helps develop health-fitness. Further, total

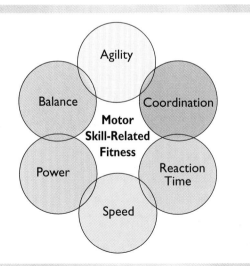

FIGURE 1.4 ✤ Motor-skill components of physical fitness.

fitness is achieved by taking part in specific programs to improve both health-related and skill-related components.

BENEFITS OF FITNESS AND WELLNESS

The benefits to be enjoyed from participating in a regular fitness and wellness program are many. In addition to a longer life (see Figures 1.5 and 1.6), the greatest benefit of all is that physically fit individuals enjoy a better quality of life. Fit people who lead a positive lifestyle live a better and healthier life. These people live life to its fullest potential and have fewer health problems than inactive individuals who also may indulge in negative lifestyle patterns.

Although compiling an all-inclusive list of the benefits reaped through participation in a fitness and wellness program is difficult, the following list summarizes many of these benefits:

1. Improves and strengthens the cardiorespiratory system.
2. Maintains better muscle tone, muscular strength, and endurance.
3. Improves muscular flexibility.

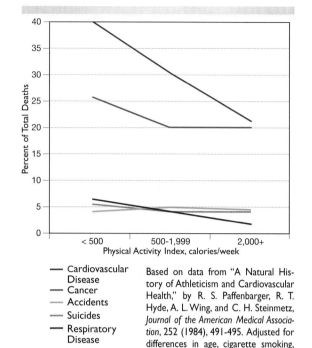

— Cardiovascular Disease
— Cancer
— Accidents
— Suicides
— Respiratory Disease

Based on data from "A Natural History of Athleticism and Cardiovascular Health," by R. S. Paffenbarger, R. T. Hyde, A. L. Wing, and C. H. Steinmetz, *Journal of the American Medical Association*, 252 (1984), 491-495. Adjusted for differences in age, cigarette smoking, and hypertension.

FIGURE 1.5 ❖ Cause-specific death rates per 10,000 man-years of observation among Harvard alumni, 1962–1978, by physical activity index.

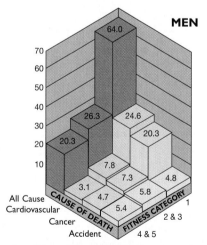

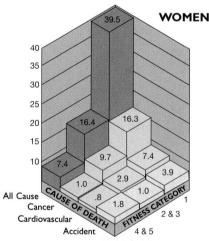

Based on data from "Physical Fitness and All-Cause Mortality: A Prospective Study of Healthy Men and Women," by S. N. Blair, H. W. Kohl III, R. S. Paffenbarger, Jr., D. G. Clark, K. H. Cooper, and L. W. Gibbons, *Journal of the American Medical Association*, 262 (1989), 2406.

FIGURE 1.6 ❖ Age-adjusted cause-specific death rates per 10,000 person-years of follow-up (1970 to 1985) in the Aerobics Center longitudinal study, Dallas, Texas.

4. Helps maintain recommended body weight.

5. Improves posture and physical appearance.

6. Decreases risk and mortality rate for chronic diseases and illness.

7. Thins the blood so it doesn't clot as readily (decreasing the risk for coronary heart disease and strokes).

8. Lowers blood pressure.

9. Helps prevent diabetes.

10. Enables people to sleep better.

11. Helps prevent chronic back pain.

12. Relieves tension and helps in coping with stresses of life.

13. Increases levels of energy and job productivity.

14. Increases longevity and slows down the aging process.

15. Improves self-image and morale and aids in fighting depression.

16. Motivates toward positive lifestyle changes.

17. Decreases recovery time following physical exertion.

18. Speeds up recovery following injury or disease.

19. Improves physical stamina and helps decrease chronic fatigue.

20. Enhances quality of life; makes people feel better and live a healthier and happier life.

In addition to the benefits listed, epidemiological research studies linking physical activity habits and mortality rates have shown lower premature mortality rates in physically active people. (Epidemiology is *the study of epidemic diseases*.) Work conducted by Dr. Ralph Paffenbarger and colleagues[8] demonstrated that as the amount of weekly physical activity increased, the risk of cardiovascular deaths decreased. In this study, conducted among 16,936 Harvard alumni, the greatest decrease in cardiovascular deaths was observed in alumni who burned more than 2,000 calories per week through physical activity (see Figure 1.5).

Another major study, conducted by Dr. Steve Blair and associates,[9] upheld the findings of the Harvard alumni study. Based on data from 13,344 people who were followed over an average of 8 years, the results confirmed that the level of cardiorespiratory fitness is related to mortality from all causes. These findings showed a graded and consistent inverse relationship between cardiorespiratory fitness and mortality, regardless of age and other risk factors. In essence, the higher the level of cardiorespiratory fitness, the longer the life (see Figure 1.6).

The death rate from all causes for the least-fit (group 1) men was 3.4 times higher than for the most fit men. For the least-fit women, the death rate was 4.6 times higher than for the most-fit women. The study also reported a greatly reduced rate of premature deaths, even at moderate fitness levels that most adults can achieve easily. People gain further protection when they combine higher fitness levels with reduction in other risk factors such as hypertension, elevated cholesterol, cigarette smoking, and excessive body fat.

Additional research that looked at changes in fitness and mortality found a substantial (44%) reduction in mortality risk when people abandon a sedentary lifestyle and become moderately fit.[10] The lowest death rate was found in people who were fit and remained fit, while the highest rate was found in men who remained unfit (see Figure 1.7).

Subsequent research published in 1995 in the *Journal of the American Medical Association*[11] substantiated the previous findings but also indicated that primarily vigorous activities are associated with greater longevity. Vigorous activity was defined as activity that requires a MET level equal to or greater than 6 METs (see Chapter 4, Table 4.1). This level represents exercising at an oxygen uptake (VO_2) equal to or greater than 21 ml/kg/min, or the equivalent of 6 times the resting energy requirement.

Examples of vigorous activities used in the previous study include brisk walking, jogging, swimming laps, squash, racquetball, tennis, and shoveling snow. Results also indicated that vigorous exercise is as important as not smoking and maintaining recommended weight.

The results of these studies clearly indicate that fitness improves wellness, quality of life, and longevity. If people are able to, vigorous exercise is preferable because it is best associated with longer life.

SURGEON GENERAL'S REPORT ON PHYSICAL ACTIVITY AND HEALTH

A landmark report on the influence of regular physical activity on health was released in July of 1996 by the U.S. Surgeon General. The significance of this historic document cannot be underestimated.

The report states that regular moderate physical activity provides substantial benefits in health and well-being for the vast majority of Americans who are not physically active. In the report, moderate physical activity has been defined as physical activity that uses 150 calories of energy per day, or 1,000 calories per week.

Among these benefits are a significant reduction in the risk of developing or dying from heart disease, diabetes, colon cancer, and high blood pressure. Regular physical activity also is important for health of muscles, bones, and joints, and it appears to reduce symptoms of depression and anxiety, improve mood, and enhance the ability to perform daily tasks throughout life. For individuals who are already moderately active, greater health benefits can be achieved by increasing the amount of physical activity.

According to the Surgeon General, improving health through physical activity is a serious public health challenge that we must meet head-on at once. More than 60% of adults do not achieve the recommended amount of physical activity, and 25% are not physically active at all. Further, almost half of all people between the ages of 12 and 21 are not vigorously active on a regular basis. This report has become a call to nationwide action. Regular moderate physical activity can prevent premature death, unnecessary illness, and disability. It can also help control health care costs and help to maintain a high quality of life into old age.

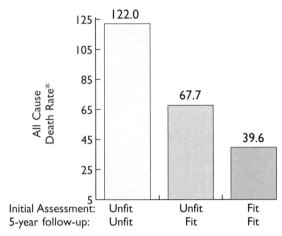

* Death rate per 10,000 man-years observation. Based on data from "Changes in Physical Fitness and All-Cause Mortality: A Prospective Study of Healthy Men," *Journal of the American Medical Association,* 273 (1995), 1193–1198.

FIGURE 1.7 ❖ Five-year follow-up in mortality rates associated with maintenance and improvements in fitness.

U. S. HEALTH OBJECTIVES FOR THE YEAR 2000

Every 10 years the U. S. Department of Health and Human Services releases a list of objectives for disease prevention and health promotion. From its onset in 1980, this 10-year plan has helped instill a new sense of purpose and focus for public health and preventive medicine.

The Year 2000 objectives, published in the document *Healthy People 2000: National Health Promotion and Disease Prevention Objectives,*[12] address three important points:

1. *Personal responsibility.* Individuals need to become ever more health-conscious. Responsible and informed behavior is the key to good health.

2. *Health benefits for all people.* Lower socioeconomic conditions and poor health often are interrelated. Extending the benefits of good health to all people is crucial to the health of the nation.

3. *Health promotion and disease prevention.* A shift from treatment to preventive techniques will drastically cut health-care costs and help Americans achieve a higher quality of life.

Development of the Year 2000 Health Objectives involved more than 10,000 people representing 300 national organizations, including the Institute of Medicine of the National Academy of Sciences, all state health departments, and the federal Office of Disease Prevention and Health Promotion. A summary of key objectives is provided in Figure 1.8. Living the fitness and wellness principles provided in this book will enhance the quality of your life and also will allow you to be an active participant in achieving the Healthy People 2000 Objectives.

THE PATH TO FITNESS AND BETTER QUALITY OF LIFE

Current scientific data and the fitness movement of the past three decades in the United States have led many people to see the advantages of participating in fitness programs that will improve and maintain adequate health. Because fitness and wellness needs vary significantly from one individual to another, all exercise and wellness prescriptions must be personalized for best results. This book provides the necessary guidelines for developing a lifetime program to improve fitness and promote preventive health care and personal wellness. As you study this book and complete the assignments in each chapter, you will learn to:

❖ Determine whether medical clearance is required for safe exercise participation.

❖ Assess your overall level of physical fitness, including cardiorespiratory endurance, muscular strength and endurance, muscular flexibility, and body composition.

❖ Prescribe personal programs for total fitness development.

❖ Write sound diet and weight control programs.

❖ Implement a healthy lifestyle program that includes prevention of cardiovascular diseases and cancer, stress management, and smoking cessation.

❖ Discern between myths and facts of exercise and health-related concepts.

MOTIVATION AND BEHAVIOR MODIFICATION

Scientific evidence of the benefits derived from living a healthy lifestyle continues to mount each day. Although the data are impressive, most people still don't adhere to a healthy lifestyle. Understanding why people do not may help increase your readiness or motivation to do so. To answer this question, one has to examine what motivates people and what actions are required to make permanent changes in behavior.

Motivation — *the desire and will to do something* — is often used as an explanation as to why some people succeed and others don't. Although motivation comes from within, external factors are what trigger the inner desire to accomplish a given task. These external factors, then, control behavior.

When studying motivation, understanding locus of control is helpful. This concept examines *the extent to which a person believes he or she can influence the external environment.* People who believe they have control over events in their lives are said to have an *internal locus of control.* People with an *external locus of control* believe that what happens to them is a result of chance, the environment, and is unrelated to their behavior.

People with an internal locus of control are healthier and have an easier time initiating and adhering to a wellness program. In contrast, those who perceive that they have no control think of themselves as powerless and vulnerable. Becoming motivated is often a challenge. These people are also at greater risk for illness. When illness strikes, restoring a sense of control is vital to regain health.

Few people have either a completely external or a completely internal locus of control. They

HEALTHY PEOPLE 2000:
SELECTED HEALTH OBJECTIVES FOR THE YEAR 2000

I. Physical Activity and Fitness

1. Increase the proportion of people who engage regularly, preferably daily, in *light* to *moderate* physical activity for at least 30 minutes per day.
2. Increase the proportion of people who engage in *vigorous* physical activity that promotes the development and maintenance of cardiorespiratory fitness 3 or more days per week for 20 or more minutes per occasion.
3. Increase the proportion of people who regularly perform physical activities that enhance and maintain muscular strength, muscular endurance, and flexibility.
4. Reduce overweight to a prevalence of no more than 20% among people aged 20 and older and no more than 15% among adolescents aged 12 through 19.

II. Nutrition

1. Reduce dietary fat intake to an average of 30% of calories or less and average saturated fat intake to less than 10% of calories among people aged 2 and older.
2. Increase complex carbohydrate and fiber-containing foods in the diets of adults to 5 or more daily servings for vegetables and fruits, and to 6 or more daily servings for grain products.
3. Increase calcium consumption in the diet.
4. Increase to at least 85% the proportion of people aged 18 and older who use food labels to make nutritious selections.

III. Chronic Diseases

1. Increase years of healthy life to at least 65 years.
2. Reduce coronary heart disease deaths.
3. Reduce the mean serum cholesterol level among adults to no more than 200 mg/dL.
4. Increase the proportion of adults with high blood cholesterol who are aware of their condition and are taking action to reduce their blood cholesterol to recommended levels.
5. Increase the proportion of people with high blood pressure whose blood pressure is under control.
6. Increase the proportion of people with high blood pressure who are taking action to help control their blood pressure.
7. Reverse the rise in cancer deaths.
8. Reduce the proportion of people who experience adverse health effects from stress.
9. Decrease the proportion of people who experience stress who do not take steps to reduce or control their stress.

IV. Tobacco

1. Reduce the incidence of cigarette smoking.
2. Reduce the proportion of children who are exposed regularly to tobacco smoke at home.
3. Reduce use of smokeless tobacco.

V. Alcohol and Other Drugs

1. Reduce the proportion of young people who have used alcohol, marijuana, and cocaine.
2. Reduce the proportion of high school seniors and college students engaging in recent occasions of heavy drinking of alcoholic beverages.
3. Reduce alcohol consumption by people aged 14 and older to an annual average of no more than 2 gallons of ethanol per person.
4. Reduce deaths caused by alcohol-related motor vehicle crashes.
5. Reduce drug-related deaths.

VI. AIDS, HIV Infection, and Sexually Transmitted Diseases

1. Confine annual incidence of diagnosed AIDS cases to no more than 98,000 cases.
2. Confine the prevalence of HIV infection to no more than 800 per 100,000 people.
3. Increase the proportion of sexually active, unmarried people who used a condom at last sexual intercourse.
4. Reduce the overall incidence of sexually transmitted diseases.

VII. Family Planning

1. Reduce the number of pregnancies that are unintended.
2. Reduce the proportion of adolescents who have engaged in sexual intercourse.
3. Increase the proportion of sexually active, unmarried people aged 19 and younger who use contraception, especially combined-method contraception that both effectively prevents pregnancy and provides barrier protection against disease.

VIII. Unintentional Injuries

1. Reduce deaths caused by unintentional injuries.
2. Increase use of occupant protection systems, such as safety belts, inflatable safety restraints, and child safety seats among motor vehicle occupants.
3. Increase use of helmets among motorcyclists and bicyclists.

* Adapted from *Healthy People 2000: National Health Promotion and Disease Prevention Objectives*, by U.S. Department of Health and Human Services (Boston: Jones and Bartlett Publishers, 1992). Refer to this publication for further information on these objectives.

FIGURE 1.8 ♣ Healthy People 2000: Selected health objectives for the year 2000.

fall somewhere along a continuum. Where a person is along the continuum relates to his or her health. Also, the more external, the greater is the challenge in adhering to exercise and other healthy lifestyle behaviors. Fortunately, developing a more internal locus of control can be accomplished. Understanding that most events in life are not genetically or environmentally controlled helps people pursue goals and gain control over their lives. Three impediments, however, can keep people from taking action:[13] competence, confidence, and motivation.

1. *Problems of competence.* Lacking the skills to get a given task done leads to decreased competence. If your friends play basketball regularly, but you don't know how to play, you might not be inclined to participate. The solution to this problem of competence is to master the skills needed to participate. Most people are not born with all-inclusive natural abilities, including playing sports.

   A college professor continuously watched a group of students play an entertaining game of basketball every Friday at noon. Having no basketball skills, he was reluctant to play. The desire to join in the fun was strong enough that he enrolled in a beginning course at the college so he would learn to play the game. To his surprise, most students were impressed that he was willing to do this. Now, with greater competence, he is able to join in on Friday's "pick-up" games.

   Another alternative is to select an activity in which you are skilled. It may not be basketball, but it could well be aerobics. Don't be afraid, however, to try new activities. Similarly, if your body weight is a problem, you could learn to cook low-fat meals. Try different recipes until you find dishes that you like.

   Patty's story at the beginning of this chapter is another example of a lack of competence. Patty was motivated and knew that she could do it, but she lacked the skills to reach her goal. Once she mastered the skills, she was able to achieve and maintain her goal.

2. *Problems of confidence.* Problems with confidence arise when the skills are there but you don't believe you can get it done. Fear and feelings of inadequacy often interfere with the ability to perform the task.

   You never should talk yourself out of something until you have given it a fair try. If the skills are there, the sky is the limit. Initially, try to visualize yourself doing the task and getting it done. Repeat this practice several times, then give it a try. You will surprise yourself.

   Sometimes lack of confidence develops when the task appears insurmountable. In these situations dividing a goal into smaller realistic objectives helps to accomplish the task. You may know how to swim, but to swim a continuous mile may take several weeks to accomplish. Set up your training program so that each day you swim a little farther until you are able to swim the entire mile. If on a particular day you don't meet your objective, try it again, reevaluate, cut back a little, and, most important, don't give up.

3. *Problems of motivation.* In problems of motivation, both the competence and the confidence are there, but the individuals are unwilling to change because the reasons for change are not important to them. For example, people begin contemplating a smoking cessation program when the reasons for quitting outweigh the reasons for smoking.

   When it comes to quality of life, lack of knowledge and lack of goals are the primary causes of unwillingness to change. Knowledge often determines goals, and goals determine motivation. How badly you want it dictates how hard you'll work at it. Many people are unaware of the magnitude of the benefits of a wellness program. Unfortunately, when it comes to a healthy lifestyle, there may not be a second chance. A stroke, a heart attack, or cancer can lead to irreparable or fatal consequences. Greater understanding of what leads to disease may be all that is needed to initiate change.

Also, feeling physically fit is difficult to explain unless you have experienced it yourself. The feelings Patty expressed to her instructor — feelings of fitness, self-esteem, confidence, health, and quality of life — cannot be conveyed to someone who is confined to sedentary living. In a way, wellness is like reaching the top of a mountain. The quietness, the clean air, the lush vegetation, the flowing water in the river, the wildlife, and the majestic valley below are difficult to explain to someone who has spent a lifetime within city limits.

BEHAVIOR MODIFICATION

Over the course of many years, we all develop habits that at some point in time we would like to change; "old habits die hard." Behavior modification — *the process to change destructive or negative behaviors permanently for positive behaviors that will lead to better health and well-being* — requires continual effort to achieve. When it comes to wellness, the sooner we implement a healthy lifestyle program, the greater are the health benefits and quality of life that lie ahead. The following principles can be adopted to help change behavior.

Self-analysis

The first step in behavior modification is a decisive desire to do so. If you have no interest in changing a behavior, you won't do it. A person who has no intention of quitting smoking will not quit, regardless of what anyone may say or how strong the evidence is against it. In your self-analysis you may want to prepare a list of reasons for continuing or discontinuing a certain behavior. As discussed earlier, when the reasons for change outweigh the reasons for not changing, you are ready for the next step.

Behavior Analysis

Determine the frequency, circumstances, and consequences of the behavior to be altered or implemented. If the desired outcome is to decrease fat consumption in the diet, you first must find out what foods in the diet are high in fat, when you eat them, and when you don't eat them. Knowing when you don't eat them points to circumstances under which you exert control of your diet and will help as you set goals.

Goal Setting

Goals motivate change in behavior. The stronger the goal (desire), the more motivated you'll be to either change unwanted behaviors or implement new healthy behaviors. The discussion on goal setting that follows will help you write goals and prepare an action plan to achieve those goals. The process will aid with behavior modification.

Social Support

Surround yourself by people who will either work toward a common goal with you or will encourage you along the way. When attempting to quit smoking, it helps to do so with others who are trying as well. You also may get help from friends who already have done so. Peer support is a strong incentive for behavioral change.

During this process, it's important also to avoid people who will not support you. Friends who have no desire to quit smoking actually may tempt you to smoke and encourage relapse of unwanted behaviors. People who are beyond the goal that you are trying to reach may not be supportive either. For instance, someone may say: "I can do six consecutive miles." Your response should be: "I'm proud that I can jog three consecutive miles."

Monitoring

Continuous behavior monitoring increases awareness of the desired outcome. Sometimes this principle by itself is sufficient to cause change. For example, keeping track of daily food intake reveals sources of fat in the diet. It can help you cut down gradually or completely eliminate high fatty foods prior to consuming them. If the goal is to increase daily fruit and vegetable intake, keeping track of the number of servings consumed each day raises awareness and may help increase their intake.

Positive Outlook

You should take a positive approach from the beginning and believe in yourself. You can do it. Following the guidelines set out in this chapter will help you pace yourself so you can work toward change. Also look at the outcomes — how much healthier you will be, how much better you will look, or being able to jog a certain distance, for instance.

Reinforcement

People tend to repeat behaviors that are rewarded and disregard those that are not rewarded or are punished. If you have been successful in cutting down fat intake during the week, reward yourself by going to a show or buying a new pair of shoes. Do not reinforce yourself with destructive behaviors such as eating a high-fat dinner. If you fail to change a desired behavior (or implement a new one), you may want to put off buying those new shoes you planned for that week. When a positive behavior becomes habitual, give yourself an even better reward. Treat yourself to a weekend away from home or go on a short trip.

GOAL SETTING

Goals are critical to initiate change. Goals motivate behavioral change and provide a plan of action. Goals are most effective when they are:

1. *Well planned*. Only a well conceived action plan will help you attain your goal. The items below, as well as others discussed in different chapters, will help you design your plan of action. You also should write specific objectives to help you reach each goal. Examples of specific objectives are provided in the Chapter 3 under "Setting Fitness Goals."

2. *Personalized*. Goals that you set for yourself are more motivational than goals someone else sets for you.

3. *Written*. An unwritten goal is simply a wish. A written goal, in essence, becomes a contract with yourself. Show this goal to a friend or an instructor and have him or her witness with their signature the contract you made with yourself.

4. *Realistic*. Goals should be within reach. If you have not exercised regularly, it would be unrealistic to start a daily exercise program consisting of 45 minutes of step aerobics at a vigorous intensity level. Unattainable goals lead to discouragement and loss of interest. To set smaller, attainable goals is better.

   At times, even with realistic goals, problems arise. Try to anticipate potential difficulties as much as possible, and plan for ways to deal with them. If your goal is to jog for 30 minutes on six consecutive days, what are the alternatives if the weather turns bad? Possible solutions are to jog in the rain, find an indoor track, jog at a different time of day when the weather improves, or participate in a different aerobic activity such as stationary cycling, swimming, or step aerobics.

5. *Measurable*. Write your goals so they are clear, and state specifically the objective to accomplish. "I will lose weight" is not clear enough and is not measurable. A better example is: "I will decrease my body fat to 17%."

6. *Time-specific*. A goal always should have a specific date for completion. This date should be realistic but not too distant in the future.

7. *Monitored*. Monitoring your progress as you move toward a goal reinforces behavior. Keeping an exercise log or doing a body composition assessment periodically determines where you are at at any given time.

8. *Evaluated*. Periodic reevaluations are vital for success. You may find that a given goal is

unreachable. If so, reassess the goal. On the other hand, if a goal is too easy, you will lose interest and may stop working toward it. Once you achieve a goal, set a new one to improve upon or maintain what you have achieved. Goals keep you motivated.

In addition to the previous guidelines, throughout this book you will find additional information on behavioral change. For example, the Exercise Readiness Questionnaire, tips to start and adhere to an exercise program, and how to set your fitness goals are provided in Chapter 3; tips to enhance your aerobic workout are given in Chapter 4; tips to adhere to a lifetime weight management program are found in Chapter 6; and a six-step smoking cessation plan and stress management techniques are provided in Chapter 7.

A WORD OF CAUTION BEFORE YOU START EXERCISE

Even though exercise testing and participation is relatively safe for most apparently healthy individuals under age 45, a small but real risk exists for exercise-induced abnormalities in people with a history of cardiovascular problems and those who are at higher risk for disease.[14] These people should be screened before initiating or increasing the intensity of an exercise program. Therefore, before you start an exercise program or participate in any exercise testing, you should fill out the health history questionnaire provided in Figure 1.9. A "yes" answer to any of these questions may signal the need for a physician's approval before you participate. If you don't have any "yes" responses, you can proceed to Chapter 2 to assess your current level of fitness.

NOTES

1. W. M. Bortz II. "Disuse and Aging." *Journal of the American Medical Association*, 248 (1982), 1203–1208.
2. Editors of *Prevention Magazine, The Prevention Index 1995: A Report Card on the Nation's Health* (Emmaus, PA: Prevention Magazine, 1995).
3. U. S. Department of Health and Human Services, National Center for Health Statistics, *Monthly Vital Statistics Report: Advance Report of Final Mortality Statistics*, 43:6, Supplement (1992), March 22, 1995.
4. T. A. Murphy and D. Murphy, *The Wellness for Life Workbook* (San Diego: Fitness Publications, 1987).
5. P. E. Allsen, J. M. Harrison, and B. Vance, *Fitness for Life* (Madison, WI: Brown & Benchmark, 1993), p. 3.
6. B. Gutin, et al., "Blood Pressure, Fitness, and Fitness in 5- and 6-Year-Old Children," *Journal of the American Medical Association*, 264 (1990), 1123–1127.

7. "Wellness Facts," *University of California at Berkeley Wellness Letter* (Palm Coast, FL: The Editors, April, 1995).
8. R. S. Paffenbarger, Jr., R. T. Hyde, A. L. Wing, and C. H. Steinmetz, "A Natural History of Athleticism and Cardiovascular Health," *Journal of the American Medical Association*, 252 (1984), 491–495.
9. S. N. Blair, H. W. Kohl III, R. S. Paffenbarger, Jr., D. G. Clark, K. H. Cooper, and L. W. Gibbons, "Physical Fitness and All-Cause Mortality: A Prospective Study of Healthy Men and Women," *Journal of the American Medical Association*, 262 (1989), 2395–2401.
10. S. N. Blair, H. W. Kohl III, C. E. Barlow, R. S. Paffenbarger, Jr., L. W. Gibbons, and C. A. Macera, "Changes in Physical Fitness and All-Cause Mortality: A Prospective Study of Healthy and Unhealthy Men,"

Journal of the American Medical Association, 273 (1995), 1193–1198.
11. I. Lee, C. Hsieh, and R. S. Paffenbarger, Jr., "Exercise Intensity and Longevity in Men: The Harvard Alumni Health Study" *Journal of the American Medical Association*, 273 (1995), 1179–1184.
12. U. S. Department of Health and Human Services, Public Health Service, *Healthy People 2000: National Health Promotion and Disease Prevention Objectives* (Boston: Jones and Bartlett Publishers, 1992).
13. G. S. Howard, D. W. Nance, and P. Myers, *Adaptive Counseling and Therapy* (San Francisco: Jossey-Bass Publishers, 1987).
14. American College of Sports Medicine, *Guidelines for Exercise Testing and Prescription* (Baltimore: Williams & Wilkins, 1995).

Health History Questionnaire

Even though exercise participation is relatively safe for most apparently healthy individuals, the reaction of the cardiovascular system to increased levels of physical activity cannot always be totally predicted. Consequently, there is a small but real risk of certain changes occurring during exercise participation. These changes include abnormal blood pressure, irregular heart rhythm, fainting, and in rare instances a heart attack or cardiac arrest. Therefore, you must provide honest answers to this questionnaire. Exercise may not be recommended under some of the conditions listed below; others may simply indicate special consideration. If any of the conditions apply, you should consult your physician before participating in an exercise program. You also should promptly report to your instructor any exercise-related abnormalities experienced during the course of the semester.

Have you ever had or do you now have any of the following conditions?

☐ Yes ☐ No 1. Cardiovascular disease (any type of heart or blood vessel disease, including strokes)

☐ Yes ☐ No 2. Elevated blood lipids (cholesterol and triglycerides)

☐ Yes ☐ No 3. Chest pain at rest or during exertion

☐ Yes ☐ No 4. Shortness of breath or other respiratory problems

☐ Yes ☐ No 5. Uneven, irregular, or skipped heartbeats (including a racing or fluttering heart)

☐ Yes ☐ No 6. Elevated blood pressure

☐ Yes ☐ No 7. Often feel faint or have spells of severe dizziness

☐ Yes ☐ No 8. Diabetes

☐ Yes ☐ No 9. Any joint, bone, or muscle problems (e.g., arthritis, low-back pain, rheumatism)

☐ Yes ☐ No 10. An eating disorder (anorexia, bulimia)

☐ Yes ☐ No 11. Any other concern regarding your ability to participate safely in an exercise program? If so, explain:

Indicate if any of the following two conditions apply:

☐ Yes ☐ No 12. Do you smoke cigarettes?

☐ Yes ☐ No 13. Men — Are you age 40 or older?

☐ Yes ☐ No 14. Women — Are you age 50 or older?

Student's Signature: _____ Date: _____

FIGURE 1.9 ✤ Health history questionnaire.

Physical Fitness Assessment

OBJECTIVES

❖ Define the health-related components of physical fitness.

❖ Be able to assess cardiorespiratory fitness, strength fitness, flexibility fitness, and body composition.

❖ Be able to determine recommended body weight.

The health-related components of physical fitness consist of cardiorespiratory endurance, muscular strength and endurance, muscular flexibility, and body composition. These four components are the topics of this chapter, along with basic techniques frequently used in their assessment. Through these assessment techniques you will be able to determine your physical fitness level regularly as you engage in an exercise program. You are encouraged to conduct fitness assessments at least twice — once as a pre-test, which will serve as a starting point, and later as a post-test, to assess improvements in fitness following 10 to 14 weeks of participation in exercise.

A personal fitness profile is provided in Appendix A, Figure A.1*, for you to record the results of each fitness assessment in this chapter (pre-test). Figure A.2 can be used at the end of the term to record the results of your post-test.

In Chapter 3 you will learn to write personal fitness goals for this course (see Figure 3.9). These goals should be based on the actual results of your initial fitness assessments. As you proceed with your exercise program, you should allow a minimum of 8 weeks before doing your post-fitness assessments.

As discussed in Chapter 1, exercise testing or exercise participation is not advised for individuals with certain medical or physical conditions. Therefore, before starting an exercise program or participating in any exercise testing, you should fill out the Health History Questionnaire given in Figure 1.9. A "yes" answer to any of the questions signals consultation with a physician before initiating, continuing, or increasing your level of physical activity.

PHYSICAL FITNESS ASSESSMENT

No single test can provide a complete measure of physical fitness. Because fitness has four different components, a battery of tests is necessary to determine an individual's overall level of fitness.

In the next few pages are several tests used to assess the health-related fitness components. When interpreting fitness test results, two standards can be applied: health fitness and physical fitness.

The health fitness or criterion referenced standards proposed here are based on epidemiological data linking minimum fitness values to disease prevention and health. These standards seem to be *the lowest fitness requirements for maintaining good health, decreasing the risk for chronic diseases, and lowering the incidence of muscular-skeletal injuries.*

Attaining the health fitness standards requires only moderate amounts of physical activity. For example, a 2-mile walk in less than 30 minutes, five to six times per week, seems to be sufficient to achieve the health-fitness standard for cardiorespiratory endurance.

Physical fitness standards are set higher than the health fitness norms and require a more vigorous exercise program. Many experts believe that people who meet the criteria of "good" physical fitness should be *able to do moderate to vigorous physical activity without undue fatigue* and to maintain this capability throughout life. In this context, physically fit people of all ages will have the freedom to enjoy most of life's daily and recreational activities to their fullest potential. Current health fitness standards may not be enough to achieve these objectives.

Sound physical fitness gives the individual a degree of independence throughout life that many people in the United States no longer enjoy. Most older people should be able to carry out activities similar to those they conducted in their youth, though not with the same intensity. Although a person does not have to be an elite athlete, activities such as changing a tire, chopping wood, climbing several flights of stairs, playing a vigorous game of basketball, mountain biking, playing soccer with grandchildren, walking several miles around a lake, and hiking through a national park require more than the current "average fitness" level of the American people.

If the main objective of the fitness program is to lower the risk for disease, attaining the health fitness standards may be enough to ensure better health. On the other hand, if the individual wants to participate in moderate to vigorous fitness activities, achieving a high physical fitness standard is recommended. For the purposes of this book, both health fitness and physical fitness standards are given for each fitness test. The individual then has to decide the personal objectives for the fitness program.

---

* You may obtain a computerized fitness profile by using the software for this book available to your instructor from Morton Publishing Company, 925 W. Kenyon, Unit 12, Englewood, CO 80110. An example of the profile is given in Figure A.3.

CARDIORESPIRATORY ENDURANCE

Cardiorespiratory endurance has been defined as *the ability of the lungs, heart, and blood vessels to deliver adequate amounts of oxygen to the cells to meet the demands of prolonged physical activity*. As a person breathes, part of the oxygen in the air is taken up in the lungs and transported in the blood to the heart. The heart then pumps the oxygenated blood through the circulatory system to all organs and tissues of the body. At the cellular level oxygen is used to convert food substrates, primarily carbohydrates and fats, into the energy necessary to conduct body functions, maintain a constant internal equilibrium, and perform physical tasks.

Some examples of activities that promote *cardiorespiratory fitness*, or aerobic fitness are walking, jogging, cycling, rowing, swimming, cross-country skiing, aerobic dance, soccer, basketball, and racquetball. The necessary guidelines to develop a lifetime cardiorespiratory endurance exercise program are given in Chapter 3, and an introduction and description of benefits of leading aerobic activities are given in Chapter 4.

A sound cardiorespiratory endurance program greatly contributes to good health. The typical American is not exactly a good role model when physical fitness is concerned. A poorly conditioned heart that has to pump more often just to keep a person alive is subject to more wear-and-tear than a well-conditioned heart is. In situations that place strenuous demands on the heart, such as doing yard work, lifting heavy objects or weights, or running to catch a bus, the unconditioned heart may not be able to sustain the strain.

Everyone who initiates a cardiorespiratory exercise program can expect a number of benefits from training. Among these are lower resting heart rate, blood pressure, blood lipids (cholesterol and triglycerides), recovery time following exercise, and risk for hypokinetic diseases (those associated with physical inactivity and sedentary living). Simultaneously, cardiac muscle strength and oxygen-carrying capacity increase.

Cardiorespiratory endurance is determined by the maximal oxygen uptake, or VO_2max, *the maximum amount of oxygen* the human body is able to utilize per minute of physical activity. The VO_2max usually is expressed in ml/kg/min. Because all tissues and organs of the body utilize oxygen to function, more oxygen consumption means a more efficient cardiorespiratory system.

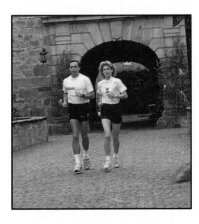
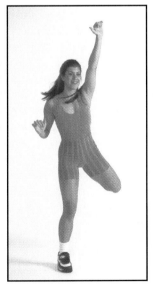
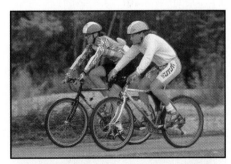
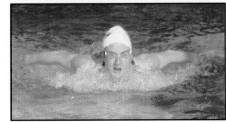

Promoting cardiorespiratory development and helping decrease the risk for chronic diseases through aerobic activities.

During physical exertion more energy is needed to perform the activity. As a result, the heart, lungs, and blood vessels have to deliver more oxygen to the cells to supply the required energy. During prolonged exercise an individual with a high level of cardiorespiratory endurance is able to deliver the required amount of oxygen to the tissues with relative ease. The cardiorespiratory system of a person with a low level of endurance has to work much harder, as the heart has to pump more often to supply the same amount of oxygen to the tissues and consequently fatigues faster. Hence, a higher capacity to deliver and utilize oxygen (oxygen uptake) indicates a more efficient cardiorespiratory system.

Even though most cardiorespiratory endurance tests probably are safe to administer to apparently healthy individuals (those with no major coronary risk factors or symptoms), the American College of Sports Medicine recommends that a physician be present for all maximal exercise tests on apparently healthy men over age 40 and women over age 50.[1] A maximal test is any test that requires the participant's

all-out or nearly all-out effort, such as the 1.5-mile run test or a maximal exercise treadmill test (stress electrocardiogram). For submaximal exercise tests (such as a walking test) a physician should be present when testing higher risk/symptomatic individuals or people with medical conditions, regardless of the participant's age.

1.5-Mile Run Test

The test used most often to determine cardiorespiratory fitness is the 1.5-Mile Run Test. The fitness category is determined according to the time a person takes to run or walk a 1.5-mile course. The only equipment necessary to conduct this test is a stopwatch and a track or premeasured 1.5-mile course.

The 1.5-Mile Run Test is quite simple to administer, but a note of caution is in order: As the objective is to cover the distance in the shortest time, it is considered a maximal exercise test. The 1.5-Mile Run Test should be limited to conditioned individuals who have been cleared for exercise. It is not recommended for unconditioned beginners, symptomatic individuals, those with known cardiovascular disease or heart disease risk factors, and men over age 40 and women over age 50. Unconditioned beginners are encouraged to have at least 6 weeks of aerobic training before they take the test.

Prior to taking the 1.5-Mile Run Test, you should do a few warm-up exercises — some stretching exercises, some walking, and slow jogging. Next, time yourself during the 1.5-Mile Run to see how fast you cover the distance. If any unusual symptoms arise during the test, do not continue. Stop immediately and see your physician or retake the test after another 6 weeks of aerobic training. At the end of the test, cool down by walking or jogging slowly for another 3 to 5 minutes. Referring to your performance time, look up your estimated VO_{2max} in Table 2.1 and the corresponding fitness category in Table 2.2.

For example, a 20-year-old female runs the 1.5-mile course in 12 minutes and 40 seconds. Table 2.1 shows a VO_{2max} of 39.8 ml/kg/min.

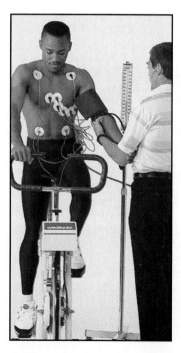

Exercise tolerance test with 12-lead electrocardiographic monitoring (stress ECG).

TABLE 2.1 ❖ Estimated Maximal Oxygen Uptake in ml/kg/min for 1.5-Mile Run Test

Time	VO$_{2max}$	Time	VO$_{2max}$	Time	VO$_{2max}$	Time	VO$_{2max}$
6:10	80.0	9:30	54.7	12:50	39.2	16:10	30.5
6:20	79.0	9:40	53.5	13:00	38.6	16:20	30.2
6:30	77.9	9:50	52.3	13:10	38.1	16:30	29.8
6:40	76.7	10:00	51.1	13:20	37.8	16:40	29.5
6:50	75.5	10:10	50.4	13:30	37.2	16:50	29.1
7:00	74.0	10:20	49.5	13:40	36.8	17:00	28.9
7:10	72.6	10:30	48.6	13:50	36.3	17:10	28.5
7:20	71.3	10:40	48.0	14:00	35.9	17:20	28.3
7:30	69.9	10:50	47.4	14:10	35.5	17:30	28.0
7:40	68.3	11:00	46.6	14:20	35.1	17:40	27.7
7:50	66.8	11:10	45.8	14:30	34.7	17:50	27.4
8:00	65.2	11:20	45.1	14:40	34.3	18:00	27.1
8:10	63.9	11:30	44.4	14:50	34.0	18:10	26.8
8:20	62.5	11:40	43.7	15:00	33.6	18:20	26.6
8:30	61.2	11:50	43.2	15:10	33.1	18:30	26.3
8:40	60.2	12:00	42.3	15:20	32.7	18:40	26.0
8:50	59.1	12:10	41.7	15:30	32.2	18:50	25.7
9:00	58.1	12:20	41.0	15:40	31.8	19:00	25.4
9:10	56.9	12:30	40.4	15:50	31.4		
9:20	55.9	12:40	39.8	16:00	30.9		

Adapted from "A Means of Assessing Maximal Oxygen Intake," by K. H. Cooper, *Journal of the American Medical Association*, 203 (1968), 201–204; *Health and Fitness Through Physical Activity*, by M. L. Pollock (New York: John Wiley and Sons, 1978); and *Training for Sport Activity*, by J. H. Wilmore (Boston: Allyn and Bacon, 1982).

TABLE 2.2 ♣ Cardiorespiratory Fitness Classification According to Maximal Oxygen Uptake in ml/kg/min

Gender	Age	Fitness Classification				
		Poor	Fair	Average	Good	Excellent
Men	≤29	≤24.9	25–33.9	34–43.9	44–52.9	≥53
	30–39	≤22.9	23–30.9	31–41.9	42–49.9	≥50
	40–49	≤19.9	20–26.9	27–38.9	39–44.9	≥45
	50–59	≤17.9	18–24.9	25–37.9	38–42.9	≥43
	60–69	≤15.9	16–22.9	23–35.9	36–40.9	≥41
Women	≤29	≤23.9	24–30.9	31–38.9	39–48.9	≥49
	30–39	≤19.9	20–27.9	28–36.9	37–44.9	≥45
	40–49	≤16.9	17–24.9	25–34.9	35–41.9	≥42
	50–59	≤14.9	15–21.9	22–33.9	34–39.9	≥40
	60–69	≤12.9	13–20.9	21–32.9	33–36.9	≥37

▨ High physical fitness standard   ▨ Health fitness or criterion referenced standard

for a time of 12:40. According to Table 2.2, this VO_{2max} places her in the good cardiorespiratory fitness category.

1.0-Mile Walk Test*

The walking test calls for a 440-yard track (four laps to a mile) or a premeasured 1.0-mile course. Body weight in pounds must be determined prior to the walk. A stopwatch is required to measure total walking time and exercise heart rate.

You can proceed to walk the one-mile course at a brisk pace so the exercise heart rate at the end of the test is above 120 beats per minute. At the end of the 1.0-Mile Walk, check your walking time and immediately count your pulse for 10 seconds. You can take your pulse on the wrist by placing two fingers over the radial artery (inside of the wrist on the side of the thumb) or over the carotid artery in the neck just below the jaw next to the voice box.

Next multiply the 10-second pulse count by 6 to obtain the exercise heart rate in beats per minute. Now convert the walking time from minutes and seconds to minute units. Each minute has 60 seconds, so the seconds are divided by 60 to obtain the fraction of a minute. For instance, a walking time of 12 minutes and 15 seconds equals 12 + (15 ÷ 60), or 12.25 minutes.

To obtain the estimated VO_{2max} in ml/kg/min. for the 1.0-Mile Walk Test, plug in your values in the following equation:

$$VO_{2max} = 132.853 - (.0769 \times W) \\ - (.3877 \times A) + (6.315 \times G) \\ - (3.2649 \times T) - (.1565 \times HR)$$

where:

W = weight in pounds
A = age in years
G = gender; use 0 for women and 1 for men
T = total time for the 1-mile walk in minutes

* "Estimation of VO_{2max} from a One-Mile Track Walk, Gender, Age, and Body Weight," by G. Kline et al., *Medicine and Science in Sports and Exercise*, 19 (3):253–259, 1987. © American College of Sports Medicine.

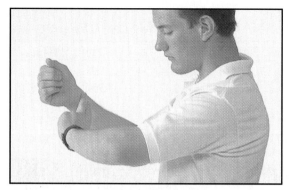

Pulse taken at the radial artery.

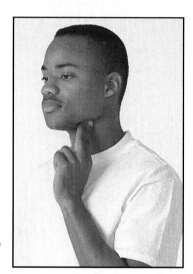

Pulse taken at the carotid artery.

HR = exercise heart rate in beats per minute at the end of the 1-mile walk

For example, a 19-year-old female who weighs 140 pounds completed the 1-mile walk in 14 minutes and 39 seconds and with an exercise heart rate of 148 beats per minute. The estimated VO_{2max} is:

W = 140 lbs
A = 19
G = 0 (female gender)
T = 14:39 = 14 + (39 ÷ 60) = 14.65 min.
HR = 148 bpm

$$\text{VO}_{2\text{max}} = 132.853 - (.0769 \times 140) - (.3877 \times 19) + (6.315 \times 0) - (3.2649 \times 14.65) - (.1565 \times 148)$$

$$\text{VO}_{2\text{max}} = 43.7 \text{ ml/kg/min.}$$

As with the 1.5-Mile Run Test, the fitness categories based on $\text{VO}_{2\text{max}}$ are found in Table 2.2. Record your cardiorespiratory fitness test results on your fitness profile in Appendix A, Figure A.1.

MUSCULAR STRENGTH/ENDURANCE

Many people are under the impression that muscular strength and endurance are necessary only for athletes and others who hold jobs that require heavy muscular work. Strength and endurance, however, are important components of total physical fitness and have become essential to everyone's life.

Adequate levels of strength significantly enhance a person's health and well-being throughout life. Strength is crucial for top performance in daily activities such as sitting, walking, running, lifting and carrying objects, doing housework, and even enjoying recreational activities. Strength is also valuable in improving personal appearance and self-image, developing sports skills, and meeting certain emergencies in life where strength is necessary to cope effectively.

Muscular strength also seems to be the most important health-related component of physical fitness in the older-adult population. Whereas proper cardiorespiratory endurance helps maintain a healthy heart, good strength levels do more toward independent living than any other fitness component.

More than anything else, older adults want to enjoy good health and function independently. Many of them, however, are confined to nursing homes because they lack sufficient strength to move about. They cannot walk very far or need to be helped in and out of beds, chairs, and tubs. A strength-training program can have a tremendous impact in enhancing quality of life.

Research has shown leg strength improvements as high as 200% in previously inactive adults over age 90.[2] As strength improves, so does the ability to move about, the capacity for independent living, and life enjoyment during the "golden years."

Perhaps one of the most significant benefits of maintaining a good strength level is its relationship to human metabolism, *all energy and material transformations that take place within living cells*. A primary result of a strength-training program is an increase in muscle mass or size, known as muscle hypertrophy.

Muscle tissue uses energy even at rest, whereas fatty tissue uses very little energy and may be considered metabolically inert from the standpoint of caloric use. As muscle size increases, so does resting metabolic rate, or the *amount of energy* (expressed in milliliters of oxygen per minute or total calories per day) *an individual requires during nonactive conditions to sustain proper body function*. Even small increases in muscle mass may affect resting metabolism.

Each additional pound of muscle tissue increases resting metabolism by an estimated 35 calories per day.[3] All other factors being equal, if two individuals who weigh 150 pounds each but have different amounts of muscle mass — let's say 5 pounds — the one with the greater muscle mass will have a higher resting metabolic rate, allowing this person to eat more calories to maintain the muscle tissue.

Although muscular strength and endurance are interrelated, the two have a basic difference. Muscular strength is *the ability to exert maximum force against resistance*. Muscular endurance (also called localized muscular endurance) is the *ability of a muscle to exert submaximal force repeatedly over a period of time*. Muscular endurance depends to a large extent on muscular strength and to a lesser extent on cardiorespiratory endurance. Weak muscles cannot repeat an action several times or sustain it for long. Keeping these concepts in mind, strength tests and training programs have been designed to measure and develop absolute muscular strength, muscular endurance, or a combination of the two.

Determining Strength

Muscular strength usually is determined by the one repetition maximum technique (1 RM), the *maximal amount of resistance a person is able to lift in a single effort*. This assessment gives a good measure of absolute strength, but it does require a considerable amount of time to administer. Muscular endurance is commonly established by the number of repetitions an individual can perform against a submaximal resistance or by the length of time a person can sustain a given contraction.

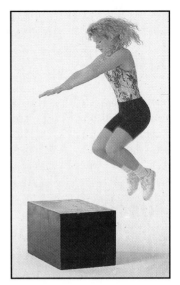

Bench jump.

Muscular Endurance Test

We live in a world in which muscular strength and endurance both are required, and muscular endurance depends to a large extent on muscular strength. Accordingly, a muscular endurance test has been selected to determine strength level. Three exercises that help assess endurance of the upper body, lower body, and abdominal muscle groups have been selected for your muscular endurance test. You will need a stopwatch, a metronome, a bench or gymnasium bleacher 16¼ inches high, and a partner to perform the test.

The exercises conducted for this test are the bench jump, modified dip (men) or modified push-up (women), and abdominal crunch. All exercises should be conducted with the aid of a partner. The correct procedures for performing these exercises follow.

Bench Jump

Using a bench or gymnasium bleacher 16¼ inches high, attempt to jump up and down on the bench as many times as you can in a 1-minute period. If you cannot jump the full minute, step up and down. A repetition is counted each time both feet return to the floor.

Modified Dip

This upper-body exercise is done by men only. Using a bench or gymnasium bleacher, place your hands on the bench with the fingers pointing forward. Have a partner hold your feet in front of you. Bend your hips at approximately 90° (you also may use three sturdy chairs; put your hands on two chairs placed by the sides of your body and your feet on the third chair in front of you).

Next, lower your body by flexing the elbows until you reach a 90° angle at this joint, and then return to the starting position. The repetition does not count if you fail to reach 90°. Perform the repetitions to a two-step cadence (down-up), regulated with a metronome set at

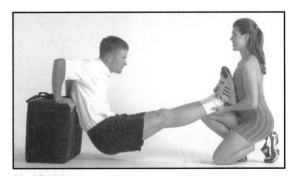

Modified-dip.

56 beats per minute. Perform as many continuous repetitions as possible. If you fail to follow the metronome cadence, you can no longer count the repetitions.

Modified Push-Up

Women perform the modified push-up exercise instead of the modified dip. Lie down on the floor (face down), bend the knees (feet up in the air), and place the hands on the floor by the shoulders with the fingers pointing forward. The lower body will be supported at the knees (rather than the feet) throughout the test. The chest must touch the floor on each repetition.

As with the modified-dip exercise, perform the repetitions to a two-step cadence (up-down) regulated with a metronome set at 56 beats per minute. Do as many continuous repetitions as possible. If you fail to follow the metronome cadence, you cannot count any more repetitions.

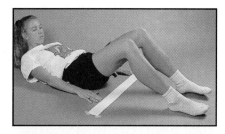

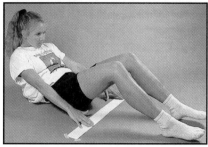

Abdominal crunch.

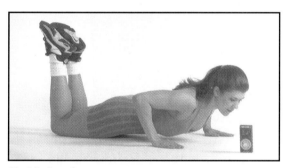

Modified push-up.

Abdominal Crunch

Tape a 3½ x 30" strip of cardboard onto the floor. Lie down on the floor in a supine position (face up) with the knees bent at approximately 100° and the legs slightly apart. The feet should be on the floor and you must hold them in place yourself throughout the test. Straighten out your arms and place them on the floor alongside the trunk with the palms down and the fingers fully extended. The fingertips of both hands should barely touch the closest edge of the cardboard. Bring the head off the floor until the chin is 1" to 2" away from your chest. Keep your head in

this position during the entire test. Do not move the head by flexing or extending the neck. You now are ready to begin the test.

Perform the repetitions to a two-step cadence (up-down) regulated with a metronome set at 60 beats per minute. As you curl up, slide your fingers over the cardboard until you feel your fingertips reach the far end (3½") of the board, then return to the starting position.

Allow a brief practice period of 5 to 10 seconds to familiarize yourself with the cadence. Initiate the up movement with the first beat and the down movement with the next beat. Accomplish one repetition every two beats of the metronome. Count as many repetitions as you are able to perform following the proper cadence. You may not count a repetition if your fingertips fail to reach the distant end of the cardboard.

Terminate the test if: (a) you fail to maintain the appropriate cadence, (b) your heels come off the floor, (c) you do not keep your chin close to the chest, (d) you accomplish 100 repetitions, or (e) you no longer can perform the test. Have your partner check the angle at the knees throughout the test to make sure the 100° angle is maintained as closely as possible.

For this test you may substitute the Crunch-Ster Curl-Up Tester, available from Novel

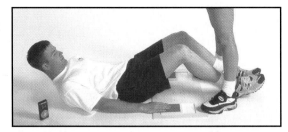

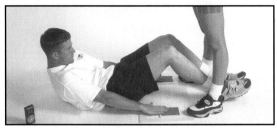

Abdominal crunch test using a Crunch-Ster Curl-Up Tester.

Products.* Because of its sliding panel, the distance traveled during each repetition is controlled carefully with this equipment.

---

*Novel Products, Inc., Figure Finder Collection, P. O. Box 408, Rockton, IL 61072–0408; 1-800-323-5143.

Interpretation of Strength Test

According to the number of repetitions performed on each test item, look up the percentile rank for each exercise in the far left column of Table 2.3. Next, total the percentile scores for each exercise and divide by 3 to obtain an average score. Determine your individual and overall muscular endurance fitness categories according to the ratings in Table 2.4.

MUSCULAR FLEXIBILITY

Muscular flexibility is the *ability of a joint to move freely through its full range of motion.* Total range of motion around a joint is highly specific and varies from one joint to the other (hip, trunk, shoulder), as well as from one individual to the next. Muscular flexibility relates primarily to genetic factors and the index of physical activity. Beyond that, factors such as joint structure, ligaments, tendons, muscles, skin, tissue injury, adipose (fat) tissue, body temperature, age, and gender influence range of motion about a joint.

TABLE 2.3 ❖ Muscular Endurance Scoring Table

Percentile Rank	MEN			WOMEN			Fitness Classification
	Bench Jumps	Modified Dips	Abdominal Crunches	Bench Jumps	Modified Push-ups	Abdominal Crunches	
99	66	54	100	58	95	100	
95	63	50	100	54	70	100	Excellent
90	62	38	100	52	50	69	
80	58	32	66	48	41	49	Good
70	57	30	45	44	38	37	
60	56	27	38	42	33	34	Average
50	54	26	33	39	30	31	
40	51	23	29	38	28	27	Fair
30	48	20	26	36	25	24	
20	47	17	22	32	21	21	Poor
10	40	11	18	28	18	15	
5	34	7	16	26	15	0	

High physical fitness standard
Health fitness or criterion referenced standard

From *Principles and Labs for Physical Fitness and Wellness,* by W. W. K. Hoeger (Englewood, CO: Morton Publishing, 1994).

TABLE 2.4 ❖ Fitness Categories Based on Percentile Ranks

Average Score	Endurance Classification
≥81	Excellent
61–80	Good
41–60	Average
21–40	Fair
≤20	Poor

High physical fitness standard

Health fitness standard (criterion referenced standard)

From *Principles and Labs for Physical Fitness and Wellness*, by W. W. K. Hoeger (Englewood, CO: Morton Publishing, 1994).

On the average, women have higher flexibility levels than men do and seem to retain this advantage throughout life. Aging decreases the extensibility of soft tissue, decreasing flexibility in both genders. The most significant contributors to loss in flexibility, however, are sedentary living and lack of physical activity.

Developing and maintaining some level of flexibility are important in all health enhancement programs, and even more so as we age. Sports medicine specialists say that many muscular/skeletal problems and injuries, especially in adults, are related to a lack of flexibility.

Most experts agree that participating in a regular flexibility program will help a person maintain good joint mobility, increase resistance to muscle injury and soreness, prevent low-back and other spinal column problems, improve and maintain good postural alignment, enhance proper and graceful body movement, improve personal appearance and self-image, and facilitate the development of motor skills throughout life. Flexibility exercises also have been used successfully in treating patients with dysmenorrhea (painful menstruation) and general neuromuscular tension. Stretching exercises in conjunction with calisthenics are helpful in warm-up routines to prepare for more vigorous aerobic or strength-training exercises, as well as subsequent cool-down routines to help return to the normal resting state.

Assessment of Flexibility

Two flexibility tests are used to determine your flexibility profile. These are the Modified Sit-and-Reach Test and the Total Body Rotation Test.

Modified Sit-and-Reach Test

To perform this test, you will need the Acuflex I* sit-and-reach flexibility tester, or you may simply place a yardstick on top of a box approximately 12" high. The procedure to administer this test is:

1. Be sure to properly warm up before the first trial.
2. Remove your shoes for the test. Sit on the floor with your hips, back, and head against a wall, legs fully extended, and the bottom of the feet against the Acuflex I or the sit-and-reach box.
3. Place the hands one on top of the other and reach forward as far as possible without letting the hips, back, or head come off the wall. Another person then should slide the reach indicator on the Acuflex I (or yardstick)

*The Acuflex I and II flexibility testers for the Modified Sit-and-Reach and the Total Body Rotation tests can be obtained from Novel Products Figure Finder Collection, P.O. Box 408, Rockton, IL 61072–0408; (800) 323–5143.

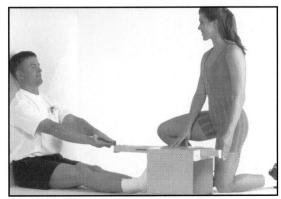

Starting position for the Modified Sit-and-Reach Test.

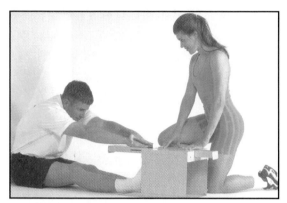
Modified Sit-and-Reach Test.

as far as possible on the indicator (or yard-stick), holding the final position for at least 2 seconds. Be sure to keep the back of the knees against the floor throughout the test. Record the final number of inches reached to the nearest half inch.

You are allowed two trials, and an average of the two scores is used as the final test score. The percentile ranks and fitness categories for this test are given in Tables 2.5 and 2.4, respectively.

Total Body Rotation Test

An Acuflex II total body rotation flexibility tester or a measuring scale with a sliding panel is needed to administer this test. The Acuflex II or scale is placed on the wall at shoulder height and should be adjustable to accommodate individual differences in height.

If an Acuflex II is not available, you can build your own scale. Glue or tape a measuring tape above the sliding panel and another below

along the top of the box until the end of the indicator touches the tips of your fingers. The indicator must then be held firmly in place throughout the rest of the test.

4. The head and back now can come off the wall, and you may reach forward gradually three times, the third time stretching forward

---

TABLE 2.5 ❖ Modified Sit-and-Reach Scoring Table

	MEN						WOMEN				
Percentile Rank	**Age Category**				**Fitness Category**	**Percentile Rank**	**Age Category**				**Fitness Category**
	<18	**19–35**	**36–49**	**>50**			**<18**	**19–35**	**36–49**	**>50**	
99	20.8	20.1	18.9	16.2		99	22.6	21.0	19.8	17.2	
95	19.6	18.9	18.2	15.8	Excellent	95	19.5	19.3	19.2	15.7	Excellent
90	18.2	17.2	16.1	15.0		90	18.7	17.9	17.4	15.0	
80	17.8	17.0	14.6	13.3	Good	80	17.8	16.7	16.2	14.2	Good
70	16.0	15.8	13.9	12.3		70	16.5	16.2	15.2	13.6	
60	15.2	15.0	13.4	11.5	Average	60	16.0	15.8	14.5	12.3	Average
50	14.5	14.4	12.6	10.2		50	15.2	14.8	13.5	11.1	
40	14.0	13.5	11.6	9.7	Fair	40	14.5	14.5	12.8	10.1	Fair
30	13.4	13.0	10.8	9.3		30	13.7	13.7	12.2	9.2	
20	11.8	11.6	9.9	8.8		20	12.6	12.6	11.0	8.3	
10	9.5	9.2	8.3	7.8	Poor	10	11.4	10.1	9.7	7.5	Poor
05	8.4	7.9	7.0	7.2		05	9.4	8.1	8.5	3.7	
01	7.2	7.0	5.1	4.0		01	6.5	2.6	2.0	1.5	

▢ High physical fitness standard

▢ Health fitness or criterion referenced standard

From *Lifetime Physical Fitness & Wellness: A Personalized Program.* by W. W. K. Hoeger (Englewood, CO: Morton Publishing, 1995.)

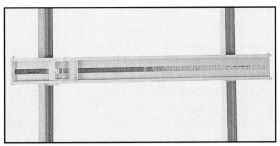

Acuflex II measuring device for the Total Body Rotation Test.

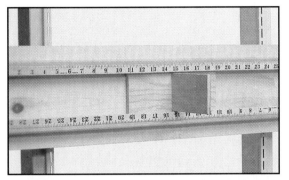

Homemade measuring device for the Total Body Rotation Test.

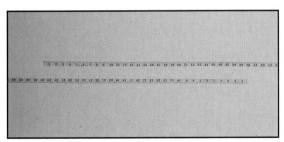

Use of measuring tapes for the Total Body Rotation Test.

it, centered at the 15" mark. Each tape should be at least 30" long. Draw a line on the floor, centered with the 15" mark. Use the following procedure:

1. Properly warm up before beginning this test.
2. To start, stand sideways, an arm's length away from the wall, with the feet straight ahead, slightly separated, and the toes right up to the corresponding line drawn on the floor. Hold out the arm opposite the wall

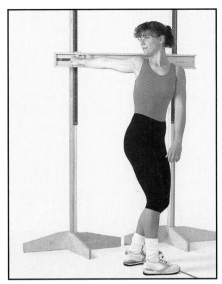

Total Body Rotation Test.

horizontally from the body, making a fist. The Acuflex II, measuring scale, or tapes should be shoulder height at this time.

3. Now rotate the body, the extended arm going backward (always maintaining a horizontal plane) and making contact with the panel, gradually sliding it forward as far as possible. If no panel is available, slide the fist alongside the tapes as far as possible. Hold the final position at least 2 seconds.

Position the hand with the little finger-side forward during the entire sliding movement. The proper hand position is crucial.

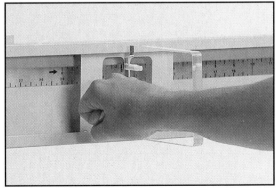

Proper hand position for the Total Body Rotation Test.

Some people attempt to open the hand or push with extended fingers or slide the panel with the knuckles, none of which is acceptable. During the test the knees can be bent slightly, but the feet cannot be moved; they always must point straight forward. The body must be kept as straight (vertical) as possible.

4. Conduct the test on either the right or the left side of the body. Two trials are allowed on the selected side. The farthest point reached, measured to the nearest half inch and held for at least 2 seconds, is recorded. The average of the two trials is the final test score. Referring to Tables 2.6 and 2.4, you can determine the respective percentile rank

TABLE 2.6 ✣ Table for Total Body Rotation Scoring

	Percentile Rank	Left Rotation Age Category				Right Rotation Age Category				Fitness Category
		<18	19–35	36–49	>50	<18	19–35	36–49	>50	
	99	29.1	28.0	26.6	21.0	28.2	27.8	25.2	22.2	
	95	26.6	24.8	24.5	20.0	25.5	25.6	23.8	20.7	Excellent
	90	25.0	23.6	23.0	17.7	24.3	24.1	22.5	19.3	
	80	22.0	22.0	21.2	15.5	22.7	22.3	21.0	16.3	
	70	20.9	20.3	20.4	14.7	21.3	20.7	18.7	15.7	Good
	60	19.9	19.3	18.7	13.9	19.8	19.0	17.3	14.7	
Men	50	18.6	18.0	16.7	12.7	19.0	17.2	16.3	12.3	Average
	40	17.0	16.8	15.3	11.7	17.3	16.3	14.7	11.5	
	30	14.9	15.0	14.8	10.3	15.1	15.0	13.3	10.7	Fair
	20	13.8	13.3	13.7	9.5	12.9	13.3	11.2	8.7	
	10	10.8	10.5	10.8	4.3	10.8	11.3	8.0	2.7	
	05	8.5	8.9	8.8	0.3	8.1	8.3	5.5	0.3	Poor
	01	3.4	1.7	5.1	0.0	6.6	2.9	2.0	0.0	
	99	29.3	28.6	27.1	23.0	29.6	29.4	27.1	21.7	
	95	26.8	24.8	25.3	21.4	27.6	25.3	25.9	19.7	Excellent
	90	25.5	23.0	23.4	20.5	25.8	23.0	21.3	19.0	
	80	23.8	21.5	20.2	19.1	23.7	20.8	19.6	17.9	
	70	21.8	20.5	18.6	17.3	22.0	19.3	17.3	16.8	Good
	60	20.5	19.3	17.7	16.0	20.8	18.0	16.5	15.6	
Women	50	19.5	18.0	16.4	14.8	19.5	17.3	14.6	14.0	Average
	40	18.5	17.2	14.8	13.7	18.3	16.0	13.1	12.8	
	30	17.1	15.7	13.6	10.0	16.3	15.2	11.7	8.5	Fair
	20	16.0	15.2	11.6	6.3	14.5	14.0	9.8	3.9	
	10	12.8	13.6	8.5	3.0	12.4	11.1	6.1	2.2	
	05	11.1	7.3	6.8	0.7	10.2	8.8	4.0	1.1	Poor
	01	8.9	5.3	4.3	0.0	8.9	3.2	2.8	0.0	

▨ High physical fitness standard
▨ Health fitness or criterion referenced standard

From *Lifetime Physical Fitness & Wellness: A Personalized Program*, by W. W. K. Hoeger (Englewood, CO: Morton Publishing Company, 1995).

and flexibility fitness classification for this test.

Interpretation of Flexibility Tests

After obtaining your score and percentile rank for both tests, you can determine your overall flexibility fitness classification by computing an average percentile rank from the two tests under the same guidelines as given in Table 2.4.

BODY COMPOSITION

Current trends indicate that, starting at age 25, the average man and woman in the United States gains 1 pound of weight per year. Thus, by age 65, the average American will have gained 40 pounds of weight. Because of the typical reduction in physical activity in our society, however, each year the average person also loses a half pound of lean tissue. Therefore, this span of 40 years has resulted in an actual fat gain of 60 pounds accompanied by a 20-pound loss of lean body mass[4] (see Figure 2.1). These changes cannot be detected unless body composition is assessed periodically.

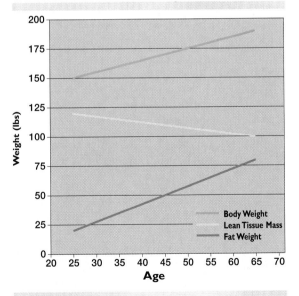

FIGURE 2.1 ❖ Typical body composition changes for adults in the United States.

Body composition refers to *the fat and non-fat components of the human body.* The *fat component of the body* usually is called fat mass or percent body fat. The *nonfat component of the body* is termed lean body mass.

Total fat in the human body is classified into two types: essential fat and storage fat. Essential fat is the *fat needed for normal physiological functions.* Without it, human health deteriorates. This essential fat constitutes about 3% of the total weight in men and 12% in women. The percentage is higher in women because it includes gender-specific fat, such as that found in the breast tissue, the uterus, and other gender-related fat deposits. Storage fat is *the fat stored in adipose tissue,* mostly beneath the skin (subcutaneous fat) and around major organs in the body.

Obesity is a health hazard of epidemic proportions in most developed countries around the world. Obesity by itself has been associated with several serious health problems and accounts for 15% to 20% of the annual U. S. mortality rate. Obesity is a major risk factor for diseases of the cardiovascular system, including coronary heart disease, hypertension, congestive heart failure, elevated blood lipids, atherosclerosis, strokes, thromboembolitic disease, varicose veins, and intermittent claudication.

Underweight people, too, have health problems and a higher mortality rate. Although the social pressure to be thin has waned slightly in recent years, pressure to attain model-like thinness is still with us and contributes to the gradual increase in eating disorders (anorexia nervosa and bulimia, discussed in Chapter 5). Extreme weight loss can spawn medical conditions such as heart damage, gastrointestinal problems, shrinkage of internal organs, immune system abnormalities, disorders of the reproductive system, loss of muscle tissue, damage to the nervous system, and even death.

For many years people relied on height/weight charts to determine recommended body weight, but we now know that these tables are highly inaccurate for many people. The standard height/weight tables, first published in 1912, were based on average weights (including shoes and clothing) for men and women who obtained life insurance policies between 1888 and 1905. The recommended weight on height/weight tables is obtained according to gender, height, and frame size. As no scientific guidelines are given to determine frame size, most people choose their frame size based on the column where the weight comes closest to their own.

The proper way to determine recommended weight is to find out what percent of total body weight is fat and what amount is lean tissue (body composition). Once the fat percentage is known, recommended body weight, the weight at which there appears to be no harm to human health, can be calculated from recommended body fat.

Obesity is related to an excess of body fat. If body weight is the only criterion, an individual easily can be considered overweight according to height/weight charts, yet not be genuinely obese. Football players, body builders, weight lifters, and other athletes with large muscle size are typical examples. Some athletes who appear to be 20 or 30 pounds overweight really have little body fat.

At the other end of the spectrum, some people who weigh very little and are viewed by many as "skinny" or underweight actually can be classified as obese because of their high body fat content. People who weigh as little as 100 pounds but are more than 30% fat (about a third of their total body weight) are not uncommon. These people are often sedentary or constantly dieting. Physical inactivity and constant negative caloric balance both lead to a loss in lean body mass (see Chapter 6). Body weight alone clearly does not always tell the true story.

Body Composition Assessment Through Skinfold Thickness

Assessment of body composition is most frequently done using skinfold thickness. This technique is based on the principle that approximately half of the body's fatty tissue is directly beneath the skin. Valid and reliable estimates of

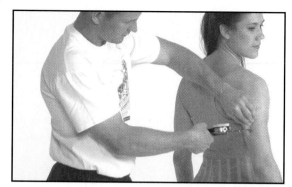

Skinfold thickness technique for body composition assessment.

this tissue give a good indication of percent body fat.

The skinfold thickness test is performed with the aid of pressure calipers. To reflect the total percentage of fat, several sites must be measured: triceps, suprailium, and thigh skinfolds for women; and chest, abdomen, and thigh for men. All measurements should be taken on the right side of the body with the person standing. The correct anatomical landmarks for skinfolds are as follows and as shown in Figure 2.2.

Chest: a diagonal fold halfway between the shoulder crease and the nipple.

Abdomen: a vertical fold about 1" to the right of the umbilicus.

Triceps: a vertical fold on the back of the upper arm, halfway between the shoulder and the arm.

Thigh: a vertical fold on the front of the thigh, midway between the knee and the hip.

Suprailium: a diagonal fold above the crest of the ilium (on the side of the hip).

Each site is measured by grasping a double thickness of skin firmly with the thumb and forefinger, pulling the fold slightly away from the muscle tissue. Hold the calipers perpendicular to the fold, and take the measurements ½" below the finger hold. Measure each site three

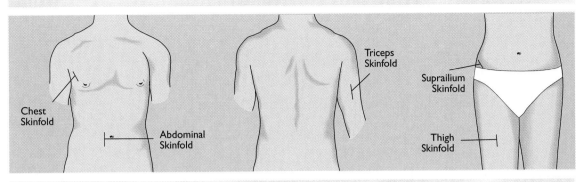

FIGURE 2.2 ❖ Anatomical landmarks for skinfolds.

times and read the values to the nearest .1 to .5 mm. Record the average of the two closest readings as the final value. Take the readings without delay to avoid excessive compression of the skinfold. Releasing and refolding the skinfold is required between readings. Be sure to wear shorts, a loose fitting t-shirt (no leotards), and do not use lotion on your skin the day when skinfolds are to be determined.

After determining the average value for each site, percent fat can be obtained by adding together all three skinfold measurements and looking up the respective values in Table 2.7 for women, Table 2.8 for men under age 40, and Table 2.9 for men over 40. Then proceed to compute your recommended body weight using the recommended percent body fat range given in Table 2.10 and the computation form in Figure 2.3.

The recommended percent body fat values given in Table 2.10 include essential fat and storage fat, previously discussed. For example, the recommended body fat range for women under age 30 is 17% to 25%. This indicates that only 5% to 13% of the total recommended fat is storage fat, and the other 12% is essential fat. The recommended range has been selected based on research indicating that some storage fat is required for optimal health and greater longevity.

The recommended body fat range selected in this book incorporates the recommendations of most health and fitness experts throughout the United States. If you desire to have just one target weight, you may select your body weight according to your personal preference, as long as it falls within the recommended range. The lower end of the range constitutes the physical fitness standard; the high end represents the health fitness standard.

Waist-to-Hip Ratio

Recent scientific evidence suggests that the way people store fat may affect the risk for disease. Some individuals have a tendency to store high amounts of fat in the abdominal area, and others store it primarily around the hips and thighs (gluteal femoral fat).

Data indicate that obese individuals with high abdominal fat are clearly at higher risk for coronary heart disease, congestive heart failure, hypertension, strokes, and diabetes than are obese people with similar amounts of total body fat that is stored primarily in the hips and thighs. Relatively new evidence also indicates that among individuals with high abdominal fat, those whose fat deposits are around internal organs (visceral fat) are at even greater risk for disease than those whose abdominal fat is primarily beneath the skin (subcutaneous fat).

Because of the increased risk for disease in individuals who tend to store high amounts of fat in the abdominal area, as opposed to the

TABLE 2.7 ✤ Percent Fat Estimates for Women Calculated from Triceps, Suprailium, and Thigh Skinfold Thickness

Sum of 3 Skinfolds	Age								
	Under 22	23 to 27	28 to 32	33 to 37	38 to 42	43 to 47	48 to 52	53 to 57	Over 58
23– 25	9.7	9.9	10.2	10.4	10.7	10.9	11.2	11.4	11.7
26– 28	11.0	11.2	11.5	11.7	12.0	12.3	12.5	12.7	13.0
29– 31	12.3	12.5	12.8	13.0	13.3	13.5	13.8	14.0	14.3
32– 34	13.6	13.8	14.0	14.3	14.5	14.8	15.0	15.3	15.5
35– 37	14.8	15.0	15.3	15.5	15.8	16.0	16.3	16.5	16.8
38– 40	16.0	16.3	16.5	16.7	17.0	17.2	17.5	17.7	18.0
41– 43	17.2	17.4	17.7	17.9	18.2	18.4	18.7	18.9	19.2
44– 46	18.3	18.6	18.8	19.1	19.3	19.6	19.8	20.1	20.3
47– 49	19.5	19.7	20.0	20.2	20.5	20.7	21.0	21.2	21.5
50– 52	20.6	20.8	21.1	21.3	21.6	21.8	22.1	22.3	22.6
53– 55	21.7	21.9	22.1	22.4	22.6	22.9	23.1	23.4	23.6
56– 58	22.7	23.0	23.2	23.4	23.7	23.9	24.2	24.4	24.7
59– 61	23.7	24.0	24.2	24.5	24.7	25.0	25.2	25.5	25.7
62– 64	24.7	25.0	25.2	25.5	25.7	26.0	26.2	26.4	26.7
65– 67	25.7	25.9	26.2	26.4	26.7	26.9	27.2	27.4	27.7
68– 70	26.6	26.9	27.1	27.4	27.6	27.9	28.1	28.4	28.6
71– 73	27.5	27.8	28.0	28.3	28.5	28.8	29.0	29.3	29.5
74– 76	28.4	28.7	28.9	29.2	29.4	29.7	29.9	30.2	30.4
77– 79	29.3	29.5	29.8	30.0	30.3	30.5	30.8	31.0	31.3
80– 82	30.1	30.4	30.6	30.9	31.1	31.4	31.6	31.9	32.1
83– 85	30.9	31.2	31.4	31.7	31.9	32.2	32.4	32.7	32.9
86– 88	31.7	32.0	32.2	32.5	32.7	32.9	33.2	33.4	33.7
89– 91	32.5	32.7	33.0	33.2	33.5	33.7	33.9	34.2	34.4
92– 94	33.2	33.4	33.7	33.9	34.2	34.4	34.7	34.9	35.2
95– 97	33.9	34.1	34.4	34.6	34.9	35.1	35.4	35.6	35.9
98–100	34.6	34.8	35.1	35.3	35.5	35.8	36.0	36.3	36.5
101–103	35.2	35.4	35.7	35.9	36.2	36.4	36.7	36.9	37.2
104–106	35.8	36.1	36.3	36.6	36.8	37.1	37.3	37.5	37.8
107–109	36.4	36.7	36.9	37.1	37.4	37.6	37.9	38.1	38.4
110–112	37.0	37.2	37.5	37.7	38.0	38.2	38.5	38.7	38.9
113–115	37.5	37.8	38.0	38.2	38.5	38.7	39.0	39.2	39.5
116–118	38.0	38.3	38.5	38.8	39.0	39.3	39.5	39.7	40.0
119–121	38.5	38.7	39.0	39.2	39.5	39.7	40.0	40.2	40.5
122–124	39.0	39.2	39.4	39.7	39.9	40.2	40.4	40.7	40.9
125–127	39.4	39.6	39.9	40.1	40.4	40.6	40.9	41.1	41.4
128–130	39.8	40.0	40.3	40.5	40.8	41.0	41.3	41.5	41.8

Body density is calculated based on the generalized equation for predicting body density of women developed by A. S. Jackson, M. L. Pollock, and A. Ward, reported in *Medicine and Science in Sports and Exercise*, 12 (1980), 175–182. Percent body fat is determined from the calculated body density using the Siri formula.

TABLE 2.8 ❖ Percent Fat Estimates for Men Under Age 40 Calculated from Chest, Abdomen, and Thigh Skinfold Thickness

Sum of 3 Skinfolds	Under 19	20 to 22	23 to 25	26 to 28	29 to 31	32 to 34	35 to 37	38 to 40
				Age				
8– 10	.9	1.3	1.6	2.0	2.3	2.7	3.0	3.3
11– 13	1.9	2.3	2.6	3.0	3.3	3.7	4.0	4.3
14– 16	2.9	3.3	3.6	3.9	4.3	4.6	5.0	5.3
17– 19	3.9	4.2	4.6	4.9	5.3	5.6	6.0	6.3
20– 22	4.8	5.2	5.5	5.9	6.2	6.6	6.9	7.3
23– 25	5.8	6.2	6.5	6.8	7.2	7.5	7.9	8.2
26– 28	6.8	7.1	7.5	7.8	8.1	8.5	8.8	9.2
29– 31	7.7	8.0	8.4	8.7	9.1	9.4	9.8	10.1
32– 34	8.6	9.0	9.3	9.7	10.0	10.4	10.7	11.1
35– 37	9.5	9.9	10.2	10.6	10.9	11.3	11.6	12.0
38– 40	10.5	10.8	11.2	11.5	11.8	12.2	12.5	12.9
41– 43	11.4	11.7	12.1	12.4	12.7	13.1	13.4	13.8
44– 46	12.2	12.6	12.9	13.3	13.6	14.0	14.3	14.7
47– 49	13.1	13.5	13.8	14.2	14.5	14.9	15.2	15.5
50– 52	14.0	14.3	14.7	15.0	15.4	15.7	16.1	16.4
53– 55	14.8	15.2	15.5	15.9	16.2	16.6	16.9	17.3
56– 58	15.7	16.0	16.4	16.7	17.1	17.4	17.8	18.1
59– 61	16.5	16.9	17.2	17.6	17.9	18.3	18.6	19.0
62– 64	17.4	17.7	18.1	18.4	18.8	19.1	19.4	19.8
65– 67	18.2	18.5	18.9	19.2	19.6	19.9	20.3	20.6
68– 70	19.0	19.3	19.7	20.0	20.4	20.7	21.1	21.4
71– 73	19.8	20.1	20.5	20.8	21.2	21.5	21.9	22.2
74– 76	20.6	20.9	21.3	21.6	22.0	22.2	22.7	23.0
77– 79	21.4	21.7	22.1	22.4	22.8	23.1	23.4	23.8
80– 82	22.1	22.5	22.8	23.2	23.5	23.9	24.2	24.6
83– 85	22.9	23.2	23.6	23.9	24.3	24.6	25.0	25.3
86– 88	23.6	24.0	24.3	24.7	25.0	25.4	25.7	26.1
89– 91	24.4	24.7	25.1	25.4	25.8	26.1	26.5	26.8
92– 94	25.1	25.5	25.8	26.2	26.5	26.9	27.2	27.5
95– 97	25.8	26.2	26.5	26.9	27.2	27.6	27.9	28.3
98–100	26.6	26.9	27.3	27.6	27.9	28.3	28.6	29.0
101–103	27.3	27.6	28.0	28.3	28.6	29.0	29.3	29.7
104–106	27.9	28.3	28.6	29.0	29.3	29.7	30.0	30.4
107–109	28.6	29.0	29.3	29.7	30.0	30.4	30.7	31.1
110–112	29.3	29.6	30.0	30.3	30.7	31.0	31.4	31.7
113–115	30.0	30.3	30.7	31.0	31.3	31.7	32.0	32.4
116–118	30.6	31.0	31.3	31.6	32.0	32.3	32.7	33.0
119–121	31.3	31.6	32.0	32.3	32.6	33.0	33.3	33.7
122–124	31.9	32.2	32.6	32.9	33.3	33.6	34.0	34.3
125–127	32.5	32.9	33.2	33.5	33.9	34.2	34.6	34.9
128–130	33.1	33.5	33.8	34.2	34.5	34.9	35.2	35.5

Body density is calculated based on the generalized equation for predicting body density of men developed by A. S. Jackson and M. L. Pollock, *British Journal of Nutrition*, 40 (1978), 497–504. Percent body fat is determined from the calculated body density using the Siri formula.

TABLE 2.9 ✤ Percent Fat Estimates for Men Over Age 40 Calculated from Chest, Abdomen, and Thigh Skinfold Thickness

Sum of 3 Skinfolds	Age							
	41 to 43	44 to 46	47 to 49	50 to 52	53 to 55	56 to 58	59 to 61	Over 62
8– 10	3.7	4.0	4.4	4.7	5.1	5.4	5.8	6.1
11– 13	4.7	5.0	5.4	5.7	6.1	6.4	6.8	7.1
14– 16	5.7	6.0	6.4	6.7	7.1	7.4	7.8	8.1
17– 19	6.7	7.0	7.4	7.7	8.1	8.4	8.7	9.1
20– 22	7.6	8.0	8.3	8.7	9.0	9.4	9.7	10.1
23– 25	8.6	8.9	9.3	9.6	10.0	10.3	10.7	11.0
26– 28	9.5	9.9	10.2	10.6	10.9	11.3	11.6	12.0
29– 31	10.5	10.8	11.2	11.5	11.9	12.2	12.6	12.9
32– 34	11.4	11.8	12.1	12.4	12.8	13.1	13.5	13.8
35– 37	12.3	12.7	13.0	13.4	13.7	14.1	14.4	14.8
38– 40	13.2	13.6	13.9	14.3	14.6	15.0	15.3	15.7
41– 43	14.1	14.5	14.8	15.2	15.5	15.9	16.2	16.6
44– 46	15.0	15.4	15.7	16.1	16.4	16.8	17.1	17.5
47– 49	15.9	16.2	16.6	16.9	17.3	17.6	18.0	18.3
50– 52	16.8	17.1	17.5	17.8	18.2	18.5	18.8	19.2
53– 55	17.6	18.0	18.3	18.7	19.0	19.4	19.7	20.1
56– 58	18.5	18.8	19.2	19.5	19.9	20.2	20.6	20.9
59– 61	19.3	19.7	20.0	20.4	20.7	21.0	21.4	21.7
62– 64	20.1	20.5	20.8	21.2	21.5	21.9	22.2	22.6
65– 67	21.0	21.3	21.7	22.0	22.4	22.7	23.0	23.4
68– 70	21.8	22.1	22.5	22.8	23.2	23.5	23.9	24.2
71– 73	22.6	22.9	23.3	23.6	24.0	24.3	24.7	25.0
74– 76	23.4	23.7	24.1	24.4	24.8	25.1	25.4	25.8
77– 79	24.1	24.5	24.8	25.2	25.5	25.9	26.2	26.6
80– 82	24.9	25.3	25.6	26.0	26.3	26.6	27.0	27.3
83– 85	25.7	26.0	26.4	26.7	27.1	27.4	27.8	28.1
86– 88	26.4	26.8	27.1	27.5	27.8	28.2	28.5	28.9
89– 91	27.2	27.5	27.9	28.2	28.6	28.9	29.2	29.6
92– 94	27.9	28.2	28.6	28.9	29.3	29.6	30.0	30.3
95– 97	28.6	29.0	29.3	29.7	30.0	30.4	30.7	31.1
98–100	29.3	29.7	30.0	30.4	30.7	31.1	31.4	31.8
101–103	30.0	30.4	30.7	31.1	31.4	31.8	32.1	32.5
104–106	30.7	31.1	31.4	31.8	32.1	32.5	32.8	33.2
107–109	31.4	31.8	32.1	32.4	32.8	33.1	33.5	33.8
110–112	32.1	32.4	32.8	33.1	33.5	33.8	34.2	34.5
113–115	32.7	33.1	33.4	33.8	34.1	34.5	34.8	35.2
116–118	33.4	33.7	34.1	34.4	34.8	35.1	35.5	35.8
119–121	34.0	34.4	34.7	35.1	35.4	35.8	36.1	36.5
122–124	34.7	35.0	35.4	35.7	36.1	36.4	36.7	37.1
125–127	35.3	35.6	36.0	36.3	36.7	37.0	37.4	37.7
128–130	35.9	36.2	36.6	36.9	37.3	37.6	38.0	38.5

Body density is calculated based on the generalized equation for predicting body density of men developed by A. S. Jackson and M. L. Pollock, *British Journal of Nutrition*, 40 (1978), 497–504. Percent body fat is determined from the calculated body density using the Siri formula.

TABLE 2.10 ❖ Recommended Body Composition According to Percent Body Fat

Age	Males	Females
≤29	12–20%	17–25%
30–49	13–21%	18–26%
≥50	14–22%	19–27%

High physical fitness standard
Health fitness or criterion referenced standard

hips and thighs, a waist-to-hip ratio test was designed by a panel of scientists appointed by the National Academy of Sciences and the Dietary Guidelines Advisory Council for the U.S. Department of Agriculture and U.S. Department of Health and Human Services. The panel recommends that men need to lose weight if the waist-to-hip ratio is 1.0 or higher. Women need to lose weight if the ratio is .85 or higher. The waist-to-hip ratio for a man with a 40" waist and a 38" hip is 1.05 (40 ÷ 38). That ratio may be indicative of increased risk for disease. Using a simple tape measure, you may determine your own waist-to-hip ratio. Record the results in Figure 2.4.

Effects of Exercise and Diet on Body Composition

If you engage in a diet/exercise program, you should repeat body composition measurements about once a month to monitor changes in lean and fat tissue. This is important because lean body mass is affected by weight reduction programs as well as physical activity. A negative

Recommended Body Weight Determination

A. Current Body Weight (BW): _____ lbs

B. Current Percent Fat (%F): _____ %

C. Fat Weight (FW) = BW × %F* = _____ × _____ = _____ lbs

D. Lean Body Mass (LBM) = BW − FW = _____ − _____ = _____ lbs

E. Age: _____

F. Recommended Fat Percent (RFP) Range (see Table 2.10):

Low End of Recommended Fat Percent Range (LRFP): _____ % (Physical Fitness Standard)

High End of Recommended Fat Percent Range (HRFP): _____ % (Health Fitness Standard)

G. Recommended Body Weight Range:

Low End of Recommended Body Weight Range (LRBW) = LBM ÷ (1.0 − LRFP*)

LRBW = _____ ÷ (1.0 − _____) = _____ lbs

High End of Recommended Body Weight Range (HRBW) = LBM ÷ (1.0 − HRFP*)

HRBW = _____ ÷ (1.0 − _____) = _____ lbs

Recommended Body Weight Range: _____ to _____ lbs

*Express percentages in decimal form (e.g., 25% = .25)

FIGURE 2.3 ❖ Recommended body weight determination.

Waist-to-Hip Ratio Computation Form

Waist (inches):   3 8

Hip (inches):   4 2

Ratio (waist ÷ hip):   _____

Recommended Standard

	Men:	<1.0
	Women:	<.85

FIGURE 2.4 ✣ Waist-to-hip ratio computation form.

caloric balance does lead to a decrease in lean body mass. These effects will be explained in detail in Chapter 6. As lean body mass changes, so will your recommended body weight.

Changes in body composition resulting from a weight control/exercise program are illustrated by a co-ed aerobics course taught during a 6-week summer term. Students participated in aerobic dance routines four times a week, 60 minutes each time. On the first and the last day of class several physiological parameters, including body composition, were assessed. Students also were given information on diet and nutrition and basically followed their own weight-control program. At the end of the 6 weeks, the average weight loss for the entire class was only 3 pounds. When body composition was assessed,

however, class members were surprised to find out that the average fat loss was actually 6 pounds, accompanied by a 3-pound increase in lean body mass (see Figure 2.5).

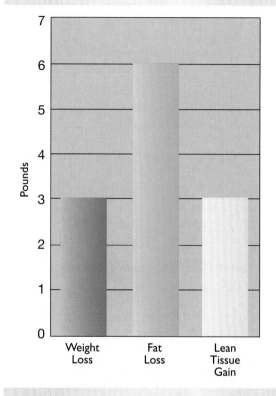

FIGURE 2.5 ✣ Effects of a 6-week aerobics program on body composition.

NOTES

1. American College of Sports Medicine, *Guidelines for Exercise Testing and Prescription* (Baltimore: Williams & Wilkins, 1995).
2. W. J. Evans, "Exercise Nutrition and Aging," *Journal of Nutrition*, 122 (1992), 786–801.
3. W. W. Campbell, M. C. Crim, V. R. Young, and W. J. Evans, "Increased Energy Requirements and Changes in Body Composition with Resistance Training in Older Adults," *American Journal of Clinical Nutrition*, 60 (1994), 167–175.
4. J. H. Wilmore. "Exercise and Weight Control: Myths, Misconceptions, Gadgets, Gimmicks, and Quackery," lecture given at annual meeting of American College of Sports Medicine, Indianapolis, June 1994.

Exercise Prescription

KEY TERMS

Aerobic exercise

Ballistic (dynamic) stretching

Cardiorespiratory training zone

Cool-down

Exercise readiness

Duration of exercise

Frequency of exercise

Intensity of exercise

Isokinetic exercise

Isometric exercise

Isotonic exercise

Mode of exercise

Overload principle

Proprioceptive neuromuscular facilitation (PNF)

Resistance

Set

Slow-sustained stretching

Specificity of training

Warm-up

OBJECTIVES

❖ Learn to write personalized cardiorespiratory, strength, and flexibility exercise programs.

❖ Be able to write fitness goals.

❖ Learn basic skills to enhance adherence to exercise.

❖ Understand biomechanical principles related to cardiorespiratory (aerobic) activities and muscular strength and endurance exercises.

A most inspiring story illustrating what fitness can do for a person's health and well-being is that of George Snell from Sandy, Utah. At age 45 Snell weighed approximately 400 pounds, his blood pressure was 220/180, he was blind because of diabetes he did not know he had, and his blood glucose (sugar) level was 487. Snell determined to do something about his physical and medical condition, so he started a walking/ jogging program. After about 8 months of conditioning, he had lost almost 200 pounds, his eyesight had returned, his glucose level was down to 67, and he was taken off medication. Two months later, less than 10 months after initiating his personal exercise program, he completed his first marathon, a running course of

26.2 miles! Research results have established that participating in a lifetime exercise program greatly contributes to good health. Nonetheless, too many individuals who exercise regularly are surprised to find, when they take a battery of fitness tests, that they are not as conditioned as they thought they were. Although these individuals may be exercising regularly, they most likely are not following the basic principles of exercise prescription. Therefore, they do not reap significant benefits.

All programs must be individualized to obtain optimal results. Our bodies are not all alike, and fitness levels and needs vary among individuals. The information presented in this chapter provides you with the necessary guidelines to write a personalized cardiorespiratory, strength, and flexibility exercise program to promote and maintain physical fitness and wellness. Information on weight control to achieve recommended body composition (the fourth component of physical fitness) is given in Chapter 6.

EXERCISE READINESS

Surveys indicate that less than 50% of the adult population in the United States exercises regularly. Further, only 20% of those who exercise are able to achieve a high physical fitness standard. Data also show that more than half of the people who start exercising drop out during the first 6 months of the program. Sports psychologists are trying to find out why some people exercise habitually and many do not. All of the benefits of exercise cannot help unless people commit to a lifetime program of physical activity.

Are you willing to give exercise a try? The first step is to decide positively that you will try. To help you make this decision, start with Figure 3.1. Make a list of the advantages and disadvantages of incorporating exercise into your lifestyle. Your list may include things such as: It will make me feel better. My self-esteem will improve. I will lose weight. I will have more energy. It will lower my risk for chronic diseases. Your list of disadvantages may include: I don't want to take the time. I'm too out of shape. There's no good place to exercise. I don't have the willpower to do it. When the reasons for exercise outweigh the reasons for not exercising, it will become easier to try.

A second questionnaire that may provide answers about your readiness to start an exercise program is provided in Figure 3.2. Carefully read each statement and circle the number that best describes your feelings. Be completely honest in your answers. You are evaluated in four categories: mastery (self-control), attitude, health, and commitment. The higher you score in any category — mastery, for example — the more important that reason is for you to exercise.

Scores can vary from 4 to 16. A score of 12 and above is a strong indicator that that factor is important to you, whereas 8 and below is low. If you score 12 or more points in each category, your chances of initiating and sticking to an exercise program are good. If you do not score at least 12 points in three categories, your chances of succeeding at exercise may be slim. You need to be better informed about the benefits of exercise, and a retraining process may be helpful. Tips on how to enhance commitment to exercise are provided later in the chapter.

CARDIORESPIRATORY ENDURANCE

A sound cardiorespiratory endurance program greatly contributes to enhancing and maintaining good health. Although health-related physical fitness has four components, cardiorespiratory endurance is the single most important fitness component, except during older age, when strength seems to be more critical. Even though certain amounts of muscular strength and flexibility are necessary for functional daily living, a person can get by without a lot of strength and flexibility but cannot do without a good cardiorespiratory system.

Principles of Cardiorespiratory Exercise Prescription

The objective of aerobic exercise is to improve the capacity of the cardiorespiratory system.

Name: _____ Date: _____

Advantages of starting an exercise program

1. _____

2. _____

3. _____

4. _____

5. _____

6. _____

7. _____

8. _____

Disadvantages of starting an exercise program

1. _____

2. _____

3. _____

4. _____

5. _____

6. _____

7. _____

8. _____

FIGURE 3.1 ❖ Advantages and disadvantages of adding exercise to your lifestyle.

To accomplish this, the heart muscle has to be overloaded like any other muscle in the human body. Just as the biceps muscle in the upper arm is developed through strength training, the *heart muscle is exercised to increase in size, strength, and efficiency.* To better understand how the cardiorespiratory system can be developed, we have to be familiar with four basic principles: intensity, mode, duration, and frequency of exercise.

The American College of Sports Medicine (ACSM) recommends that a medical exam and a diagnostic exercise stress test be administered prior to vigorous exercise by apparently healthy men over age 40 and women over 50.[1] ACSM has defined "vigorous exercise" as an exercise intensity that provides a "substantial challenge" to the participant or one that cannot be maintained for 20 continuous minutes.

Intensity of Exercise

Intensity refers to *how hard a person has to exercise to improve cardiorespiratory endurance.* Muscles have to be overloaded for them to

Name: _____ Date: _____

Carefully read each statement and circle the number that best describes your feelings in each statement. Please be completely honest with your answers.

	Strongly Agree	Mildly Agree	Mildly Disagree	Strongly Disagree
1. I can walk, ride a bike (or a wheelchair), swim, or walk in a shallow pool.	④	3	2	1
2. I enjoy exercise.	4	③	2	1
3. I believe exercise can help decrease the risk for disease and premature mortality.	④	3	2	1
4. I believe exercise contributes to better health.	④	3	2	1
5. I have previously participated in an exercise program.	4	③	2	1
6. I have experienced the feeling of being physically fit.	④	3	2	1
7. I can envision myself exercising.	④	3	2	1
8. I am contemplating an exercise program.	④	3	2	1
9. I am willing to stop contemplating and give exercise a try for a few weeks.	④	3	2	1
10. I am willing to set aside time at least three times a week for exercise.	④	3	2	1
11. I can find a place to exercise (the streets, a park, a YMCA, a health club).	④	3	2	1
12. I can find other people who would like to exercise with me.	4	③	2	1
13. I will exercise when I am moody, fatigued, and even when the weather is bad.	④	3	2	1
14. I am willing to spend a small amount of money for adequate exercise clothing (shoes, shorts, leotards, or swimsuit).	④	3	2	1
15. If I have any doubts about my present state of health, I will see a physician before beginning an exercise program.	④	3	2	1
16. Exercise will make me feel better and improve my quality of life.	④	3	2	1

Scoring Your Test:

This questionnaire allows you to examine your readiness for exercise. You have been evaluated in four categories: mastery (self-control), attitude, health, and commitment. Mastery indicates that you can be in control of your exercise program. Attitude examines your mental disposition toward exercise. Health provides evidence of the wellness benefits of exercise. Commitment shows dedication and resolution to carry out the exercise program. Write the number you circled after each statement in the corresponding spaces below. Add the scores on each line to get your totals. Scores can vary from 4 to 16. A score of 12 and above is a strong indicator that that factor is important to you, and 8 and below is low. If you score 12 or more points in each category, your chances of initiating and adhering to an exercise program are good. If you fail to score at least 12 points in three categories, your chances of succeeding at exercise may be slim. You need to be better informed about the benefits of exercise, and a retraining process may be required.

Mastery: 1. __4__ + 5. __3__ + 6. __4__ + 9. __4__ = __15__

Attitude: 2. __3__ + 7. __4__ + 8. __4__ + 13. __4__ = __15__

Health: 3. __4__ + 4. __4__ + 15. __4__ + 16. __4__ = __16__

Commitment: 10. __4__ + 11. __4__ + 12. __3__ + 14. __4__ = __15__

FIGURE 3.2 ❖ Exercise readiness questionnaire.

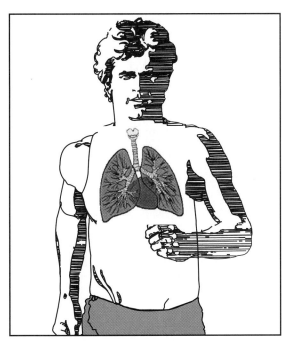

Cardiorespiratory endurance — ability of the heart, lungs, and blood vessels to deliver adequate amounts of oxygen to the cells to meet the demands of prolonged physical activity.

develop. While the training stimulus to develop the biceps muscle can be accomplished with curl-up exercises, the stimulus for the cardiorespiratory system is provided by making the heart pump at a higher rate for a certain period of time.

Cardiorespiratory development occurs when the heart is working between 50% and 85% of heart rate reserve. Increases in maximal oxygen uptake (VO_{2max}) are accelerated when the heart is working closer to 85% of heart rate reserve. For this reason, many experts prescribe exercise between 70% and 85% for young people. Exercise intensity can be calculated easily, and training can be monitored by checking your pulse. To determine the intensity of exercise or cardiorespiratory training zone, follow these steps:

1. Estimate your maximal heart rate (MHR) according to the following formula:

   MHR = 220 minus age (220 − age)

2. Check your resting heart rate (RHR) some time after you have been sitting quietly for 15 to 20 minutes. You may take your pulse for 30 seconds and multiply by 2, or take it for a full minute. As explained in Chapter 2, you can check your pulse on the wrist by placing two or three fingers over the radial artery or over the carotid artery in the neck.

3. Determine the heart rate reserve (HRR) by subtracting the resting heart rate from the maximal heart rate (HRR = MHR − RHR).

4. Calculate the training intensities (TI) at 50%, 70%, and 85%. Multiply the heart rate reserve by the respective 50, 70, and 85 percentages, and then add the resting heart rate to all three of these figures (for example, 85% TI = HRR × .85 + RHR).

   Example. The 50, 70, and 85 percent training intensities for a 20-year-old with a resting heart rate of 68 beats per minute (bpm) would be:

   MHR: 220 − 20 = 200 bpm
   RHR = 68 bpm
   HRR: 200 − 68 = 132 beats
   50% TI = (132 × .50) + 68 = 134 bpm
   70% TI = (132 × .70) + 68 = 160 bpm
   85% TI = (132 × .85) + 68 = 180 bpm
   Cardiorespiratory training zone: 134 to 180 bpm

The cardiorespiratory training zone is the *range of intensity at which a person should exercise to develop the cardiorespiratory system.* When you exercise to improve the cardiorespiratory system, you should maintain the heart rate between the 50% and 85% training intensities to obtain adequate development. If you have been physically inactive, you should train around the 50% intensity during the first 4 to 6 weeks of the exercise program. After the first few weeks, you should exercise between 70% and 85% training intensity.

Following a few weeks of training, you may have a considerably lower resting heart rate (10 to 20 beats fewer in 8 to 12 weeks). Therefore, you should recompute your target zone periodically. You can compute your own cardiorespiratory training zone by using the form in Figure 3.3. Once you have reached an ideal level of cardiorespiratory endurance, training in the 50% to 85% range will allow you to maintain your fitness level.

To develop the cardiorespiratory system, you do not have to exercise above the 85% rate. From a fitness standpoint, training above this percentage will not give extra benefits and may actually be unsafe for some individuals. For unconditioned people and older adults, cardiorespiratory training should be conducted around the 50% rate to discourage potential problems associated with high-intensity exercise.

Mode of Exercise

The mode of exercise, the *type of exercise with respect to outcome*, to develop the cardiorespiratory system has to be aerobic in nature. Aerobic exercise involves the major muscle groups of the body, and it has to be rhythmic and continuous. As the amount of muscle mass involved during exercise increases, so does the effectiveness of the activity in providing cardiorespiratory development.

Once you have established your cardiorespiratory training zone, any activity or combination of activities that will get your heart rate up to that training zone and keep it there for as long as you exercise will give you adequate development. Examples of these activities are walking, jogging, aerobics, swimming, water aerobics, cross-country skiing, rope skipping, cycling, racquetball, stair climbing, and stationary running or cycling.

The activity you choose should be based on your personal preferences, what you most enjoy doing, and your physical limitations. The amount of strength or flexibility you develop through various activities differs, but in terms of cardiorespiratory development, the heart doesn't know whether you are walking, swimming, or cycling. All the heart knows is that it has to pump at a certain rate, and as long as that rate

is in the desired range, your cardiorespiratory fitness will improve.

From a health fitness point of view, training in the lower end of the cardiorespiratory zone will yield optimal health benefits. The closer the heart rate is to the higher end of the cardiorespiratory training zone, however, the greater will be the improvements in VO_{2max} (high physical fitness).

Duration of Exercise

In terms of duration of exercise, or *time exercising per session*, the general recommendation is that a person train between 20 and 60 minutes per session. The duration is based on how intensely a person trains. If the training is done around 85%, 20 minutes are sufficient. At 50% intensity the person should train at least 30 minutes. As mentioned in the discussion of intensity of exercise, unconditioned people and older adults should train at lower percentages; therefore, the activity should be carried out over a longer time.

Although most experts recommend 20 to 30 minutes of aerobic exercise per session, 1990 research published in the *American Journal of Cardiology* indicates that three 10-minute exercise sessions per day (separated by at least 4 hours), at approximately 70% of maximal heart rate, also produce training benefits.[2] Although the increases in VO_{2max} with this program were not as large (57%) as those in a group performing one continuous 30-minute bout of exercise per day, the researchers concluded that moderate-intensity exercise training, conducted for 10 minutes three times per day, benefits the cardiorespiratory system significantly.

Results of this study are meaningful because people often mention lack of time as the reason for not taking part in an exercise program. Many think they have to exercise at least 20 continuous minutes to get any benefits at all. Even though 20 to 30 minutes are recommended, short, intermittent exercise bouts also are helpful to the cardiorespiratory system.

Exercise sessions always should be preceded by a 5-minute warm-up and followed by a

muscle cells are overloaded beyond their normal use, such as in strength-training programs, the cells increase in size (hypertrophy), strength, or endurance, or some combination of these. If the demands on the muscle cells decrease, such as in sedentary living or required rest because of illness or injury, the cells decrease in size (atrophy) and lose strength.

Overload Principle

The overload principle states that *for strength or endurance to improve, the demands placed on the muscle must be increased systematically and progressively over time, and the resistance (weight lifted) must be of a magnitude significant enough to cause physiologic adaptation.* In simpler terms, just like all other organs and systems of the human body, *muscles have to be taxed beyond their regular accustomed loads to increase in physical capacity.*

Specificity of Training

Muscular strength is the ability to exert maximum force against resistance. Muscular endurance (also referred to as localized muscular endurance) is the ability of a muscle to exert submaximal force repeatedly over a period of time.

The principle of specificity of training states that *for a muscle to increase in strength or endurance, the training program must be specific to obtain the desired effects.* As discussed later in this section, a person attempting to increase muscular strength needs a program of few repetitions and near maximum resistance. To increase muscular endurance, the strength-training program consists primarily of many repetitions at a lower resistance.

In like manner, to increase isometric (static) versus isotonic (dynamic) strength (see mode of training, below) an individual must use the corresponding static or dynamic training procedures to achieve the appropriate results. If a person is trying to improve a specific movement or skill through strength gains, the selected strength-training exercises must resemble the actual movement or skill as closely as possible.

Principles of Strength-Training Prescription

Similar to the prescription of cardiorespiratory exercise, several principles have to be observed to improve muscular strength and endurance. These principles relate to mode, resistance, sets, and frequency of training.

Mode of Training

Two basic training methods are used to improve strength: isometric and isotonic. In isometric exercise, such as pushing or pulling against immovable objects, a *muscle contraction produces little or no movement.* In isotonic exercise, a *muscle contraction is accompanied by movement*, such as lifting an object over the head.

Isometric training does not require much equipment. It was used commonly several years ago, but its popularity has waned. Because strength gains with isometric training are specific to the angle of muscle contraction, this type of training is beneficial in a sport such as gymnastics, which requires regular static contractions during routines.

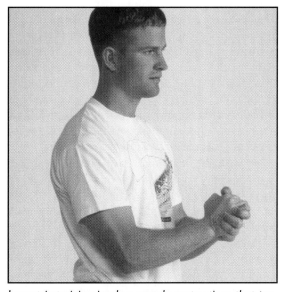

Isometric training: involves muscle contractions that produces little or no movement.

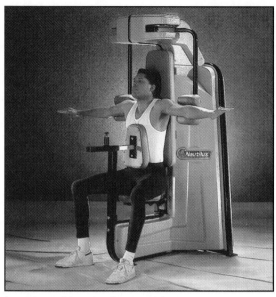

Isotonic training: involves muscle contractions accompanied by movement.

Isotonic training can be conducted without weights or with free weights (barbells and dumbbells), fixed-resistance machines, variable-resistance machines, and isokinetic equipment. When performing isotonic exercises without weights (for example, pull-ups, push-ups), with free weights, or with fixed resistance machines, a constant resistance (weight) is moved through a joint's full range of motion. The greatest resistance that can be lifted equals the maximum weight that can be moved at the weakest angle of the joint, because of changes in muscle length and angle of pull as the joint moves through its range of motion.

As strength training became more popular, new strength-training machines were developed. This technology brought about isokinetic and variable-resistance training. These training programs require special machines equipped with mechanical devices that provide differing amounts of resistance, with the intent of overloading the muscle group maximally through the entire range of motion. A distinction of isokinetic exercise is that the *speed of the muscle contraction is kept constant because the machine provides resistance to match the user's force through the range of motion.* Because of the expense of the equipment needed for isokinetic training, this type of program usually is reserved for clinical settings (physical therapy), research laboratories, and professional sports.

The mode of training depends mainly on the type of equipment available and the specific objective of the training program. Isotonic training is the most popular mode for strength training. Its primary advantage is that strength is gained through the full range of motion. Most daily activities are isotonic. We are constantly lifting, pushing, and pulling objects, which requires strength through a complete range of motion. Another advantage is that improvements are measured easily by the amount lifted.

The benefits of isokinetic and variable-resistance training are similar to those of the other isotonic training methods. Theoretically, strength gains should be better because maximum resistance is applied through the entire range of motion. Research, however, has not shown this type of training to be more effective than other modes of isotonic training. A possible advantage is that specific speeds in various sport skills can be duplicated more closely with isokinetic strength training, which may enhance performance (specificity of training). A disadvantage is

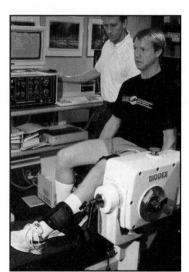

Isokinetic training requires specialized equipment.

Courtesy of Idaho Sports Medicine Institute, Boise, Idaho.

that the equipment is not readily available to everyone.

Resistance

Resistance in strength training is the equivalent of intensity in cardiorespiratory exercise prescription. The resistance, or *amount of weight lifted*, depends on whether the individual is trying to develop muscular strength or muscular endurance.

To stimulate strength development, a resistance of approximately 80% of the maximum capacity is recommended. For example, a person whose one repetition maximum (1 RM) for a given exercise is 150 pounds should work with at least 120 pounds (150 × .80). Using less than 80% will foster muscular endurance rather than strength. The time factor involved in constantly determining the 1 RM on each lift to ensure working above 80% is prohibitive. Therefore, a rule of thumb widely accepted by many authors and coaches is that *individuals should perform between 3 and 12 repetitions maximum (3 to 12 RM) for adequate strength gains.*

For example, if a person is training with a resistance of 120 pounds and cannot lift it more than 12 times, the training stimulus is adequate for strength development. Once the person can lift this resistance more than 12 times, the resistance should be increased by 5 to 10 pounds and the person again should build up to 12 RM. Training with more than 12 repetitions develops muscular endurance primarily. A person training with 20 maximum or near maximum repetitions, for example, will experience incremental increases in localized muscular endurance (localized to the specific muscle groups involved in the exercise).

Strength research indicates that the closer a person trains to the 1 RM, the greater are the strength gains. A disadvantage of working constantly at or near the 1 RM is that it increases the risk for injury. Highly trained athletes seeking maximum strength development do 1 to 6 RM. Working around 10 RM seems to produce the best results in terms of muscular hypertrophy.

Body builders tend to work with moderate resistance levels (60% to 85% of the 1 RM) and perform 8 to 20 repetitions to near fatigue. A foremost objective of body building is to increase muscle size. Moderate resistance promotes blood flow to the muscles, "pumping up the muscles" (also known as "the pump") and making them look much larger than they are in a relaxed state.

From a health-fitness point of view, 6 to 12 RM are ideal. We live in an "isotonic world" in which muscular strength and endurance both are required to lead an enjoyable life. Therefore, working near a 10 RM threshold seems best to improve overall performance.

Sets

A set in strength training has been defined as *the number of repetitions performed for a given exercise*. For example, a person lifting 120 pounds eight times performs one set of eight repetitions (1 × 8 × 120). The number of sets recommended for optimum development is three sets per exercise.

When working with 8 to 12 repetitions maximum, three sets per exercise are recommended. Because of the characteristics of muscle fiber, the number of sets that can be done is limited. As the number of sets increases, so does the amount of muscle fatigue and subsequent recovery time; therefore, strength gains may be lessened by performing too many sets.

A recommended program for beginners in their first year of training is three heavy sets, up to the maximum number of repetitions, preceded by one or two light warm-up sets using about 50% of the 1 RM (no warm-up sets are necessary for subsequent exercises that use the same muscle group). Because of the lower resistances used in body building, four to eight sets can be done for each exercise.

To make the exercise program more time-effective, two or three exercises that require different muscle groups may be alternated. In this way, a person will not have to wait 2 to 3 minutes before proceeding to a new set on a different exercise. For example, bench presses, leg extensions, and abdominal crunches may be combined so the person can go almost directly from one set to the next. Body builders should rest no more than a minute to maximize the "pumping" effect.

To avoid muscle soreness and stiffness, new participants ought to build up gradually to the three sets of maximal repetitions. This can be done by performing only one set of each exercise with a lighter resistance on the first day. During the second session, two sets of each exercise can be done, one light and the second with the regular resistance. During the third session, three sets could be performed, one light and two heavy ones. After that, a person should be able to do all three heavy sets.

Frequency of Training

Strength training should be done either with a total body workout three times per week, or more frequently if using a split-body routine (upper body one day and lower body the next). After a maximum strength workout, the muscles should be rested for about 48 hours to allow adequate recovery. If not completely recovered in 2 or 3 days, the person is most likely overtraining and therefore not reaping the full benefits of the program. In that case, a decrease in the total number of sets or exercises, or both, performed during the previous workout is recommended. A summary of strength training guidelines for health-fitness purposes is provided in Figure 3.5.

To achieve significant strength gains, a minimum of 8 weeks of consecutive training is needed. Once an ideal level of strength is achieved, one training session per week will be sufficient to maintain the new strength level.

Frequency of strength training for body builders varies from person to person. Because they use moderate resistances, daily or even two-a-day workouts are common. The frequency depends on the amount of resistance, number of sets performed per session, and the person's ability to recover from the previous exercise bout (see Table 3.1). The latter often is dictated by level of conditioning.

Mode:	8 to 10 isotonic strength-training exercises involving the body's major muscle groups
Resistance:	Enough resistance to perform 8 to 12 repetitions to near fatigue
Sets:	A minimum of 1 set
Frequency:	At least two times per week

Based on the recommended quantity and quality of exercise for developing and maintaining cardiorespiratory and muscular fitness in healthy adults by the American College of Sports Medicine, *Medical Science Sports Exercise*, 22, (1990), 265–274.

FIGURE 3.5 ❖ Strength-training guidelines.

Designing Your Own Strength-Training Program

Two strength-training programs, presented in Appendix B, have been developed to provide a complete body workout. Only a minimum of equipment is required for the first program, "Strength-Training Exercises Without Weights" (Exercises 1 through 10). This program can be

TABLE 3.1 ❖ Guidelines for Various Strength Training Programs

Strength Training Program	Resistance	Sets	Rest Between Sets*	Frequency (workouts per week)**
Health fitness	8–12 reps max	3	2 min	2–3
Maximal strength	1–6 reps max	3–6	3 min	2–3
Muscular endurance	10–30 reps	3–6	2 min	3–6
Body building	8–20 reps near max	3–8	0–1 min	4–12

* Recovery between sets can be decreased by alternating exercises that use different muscle groups.
** Weekly training sessions can be increased by using a split body routine.

conducted within the walls of your own home. Your body weight is used as the primary resistance for most exercises. A few exercises call for a friend's help or basic implements from around your home to provide greater resistance. The second program, "Strength-Training Exercises With Weights" (Exercises 11 through 17), require machines such as those shown in the various photographs. Many of these exercises also can be performed with free weights.

Depending on the facilities available to you, choose one of the two training programs outlined in Appendix B. The resistance and the number of repetitions you use should be based on whether you want to increase muscular strength or muscular endurance. Do up to 12 RM for strength gains and more than 12 for muscular endurance. As pointed out, three training sessions per week on nonconsecutive days is an ideal arrangement for proper development. Because both strength and endurance are required in daily activities, three sets of about 12 RM for each exercise are recommended. In doing this, you will obtain good strength gains and yet be close to the endurance threshold.

Perhaps the only exercise that calls for more than 12 repetitions is the abdominal group of exercises. The abdominal muscles are considered primarily antigravity or postural muscles. Hence, a little more endurance may be required. When doing abdominal work, about 20 repetitions per set are recommended. Once you begin your strength-training program, you may use the form provided in Figure 3.11 at the end of this chapter to keep a record of your training sessions.

If time is a concern in completing a strength-training exercise program, the American College of Sports Medicine recommends a minimum of one set of 8 to 12 repetitions performed to near fatigue, using 8 to 10 exercises that involve the major muscle groups of the body[4] (see Figure 3.12 at the end of this chapter). Training sessions should be conducted twice a week (see Figure 3.5). The recommendation is based on research showing that this training generates 70% to 80% of the improvements reported in other programs using three sets of about 10 RM.

MUSCULAR FLEXIBILITY

Improving and maintaining good joint range of motion throughout life is important in enhancing health and quality of life. Nevertheless, health care professionals and practitioners generally have underestimated and overlooked flexibility fitness.

The most significant detriments to flexibility are sedentary living and lack of physical activity. As physical activity decreases, muscles lose elasticity and tendons and ligaments tighten and shorten. Aging also reduces the extensibility of soft tissue, decreasing flexibility.

Generally, flexibility exercises to improve joint range of motion are conducted following an aerobic workout. Stretching exercises seem to be most effective when a person is warmed up properly. Cool muscle temperatures decrease joint range of motion. Changes in muscle temperature can increase or decrease flexibility by as much as 20%. Because of the effects of muscular temperature on flexibility, many people prefer to do their stretching exercises after the aerobic phase of their workout.

Principles of Muscular Flexibility Prescription

The overload and specificity of training principles also apply to development of muscular flexibility. To increase the total range of motion of a joint, the specific muscles surrounding that joint have to be stretched progressively beyond their accustomed length. The principles of mode, intensity, repetitions, and frequency of exercise also can be applied to flexibility programs.

Mode of Exercise

Three modes of stretching exercises promote flexibility:

1. Ballistic stretching.
2. Slow-sustained stretching.
3. Proprioceptive neuromuscular facilitation stretching.

Although all three types of stretching are effective in developing better flexibility, each has certain advantages.

Ballistic or dynamic stretching exercises require *jerky, rapid, and bouncy movements that provide the necessary force to lengthen the muscles.* This type of stretching helps to develop flexibility, but the ballistic actions may cause muscle soreness and injury because of small tears to the soft tissue.

Precautions must be taken not to overstretch ligaments, because they undergo plastic (permanent) elongation. If the stretching force cannot be controlled, as in fast, jerky movements, ligaments can be overstretched easily. This, in turn, leads to excessively loose joints, increasing the risk for injuries, including joint dislocation and subluxation (partial dislocation). Most authorities, therefore, do not recommend ballistic exercises for development of flexibility.

With the slow-sustained stretching technique, *muscles are lengthened gradually through a joint's complete range of motion, and the final position is held for a few seconds.* Doing a slow-sustained stretch causes the muscles to relax so greater length can be achieved. This type of stretch causes little pain and has a low risk of injury. Slow-sustained stretching exercises are the most frequently used and recommended for flexibility development programs.

Proprioceptive neuromuscular facilitation (PNF) stretching has become more popular in the last few years. This technique, *based on a "contract and relax" method,* requires the assistance of another person. The procedure is as follows:

1. The person assisting with the exercise provides initial force by pushing slowly in the direction of the desired stretch. The initial stretch does not cover the entire range of motion.

2. The person being stretched then applies force in the opposite direction of the stretch, against the assistant, who tries to hold the initial degree of stretch as closely as possible. An isometric contraction is being performed at that angle.

3. After 4 or 5 seconds of isometric contraction, the muscles being stretched are relaxed completely. The assistant then increases the degree of stretch slowly to a greater angle.

4. The isometric contraction is repeated for another 4 or 5 seconds; then the muscle(s) is relaxed again. The assistant then can slowly increase the degree of stretch one more time.

This procedure is repeated two to five times, until the exerciser feels mild discomfort. On the last trial the final stretched position should be held several seconds.

Theoretically, with the PNF technique, the isometric contraction helps relax the muscle(s) being stretched, which results in greater muscle length. Some fitness leaders believe PNF is more effective than slow-sustained stretching. Another benefit of PNF is an increase in strength of the

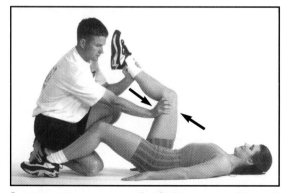
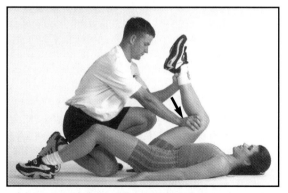

Proprioceptive neuromuscular facilitation stretching technique (a) isometric phase (b) stretching phase.

muscle(s) being stretched. Recent research showed an approximate 17% and 35% increase in absolute strength and muscular endurance, respectively, in the hamstring muscle group through 12 weeks of PNF stretching.[5] The results were consistent in both men and women. These increases are attributed to the isometric contractions performed during PNF. The disadvantages are more pain with PNF, a second person is required to assist, and more time is needed to conduct each session.

Intensity of Exercise

The intensity, or degree of stretch, when doing flexibility exercises should be only *to a point of mild discomfort*. Pain does not have to be part of the stretching routine. Excessive pain is an indication that the load is too high and may lead to injury.

All stretching should be done to slightly below the pain threshold. As participants reach this point, they should try to relax the muscle being stretched as much as possible. After completing the stretch, the body part is brought back gradually to the starting point.

Repetitions

The time required for an exercise session for development of flexibility is based on the number of repetitions performed and the length of time each repetition (final stretched position) is held. The general recommendation is that each exercise be done four or five times, holding the final position each time for about 10 to 20 seconds.

As flexibility increases, a person can gradually increase the time each repetition is held, to a maximum of 1 minute. Individuals who are susceptible to flexibility injuries should limit each stretch to 20 seconds.

Frequency of Exercise

In the early stages of the program, flexibility exercises should be conducted five to six times a week. After a minimum of 6 to 8 weeks of almost daily stretching, flexibility levels can be maintained with only two or three sessions per week, using about three repetitions of 10 to 15 seconds each. Figure 3.6 provides a summary of flexibility development guidelines.

When To Stretch?

Many people do not differentiate a warm-up from stretching. Warming up means starting a workout slowly with walking, slow jogging, or light calisthenics. Stretching implies movement of joints through their range of motion.

Before performing flexibility exercises, the muscles should be warmed up properly. Failing to warm up increases the risk for muscle pulls and tears. Surveys have shown that individuals who stretch before workouts without an adequate warm-up actually have a higher rate of injuries than those who do not stretch at all.

A good time to do flexibility exercises is after aerobic workouts. Higher body temperature in itself helps to increase joint range of motion. Muscles also are fatigued following exercise. A fatigued muscle tends to shorten, which can lead to soreness and spasms. Stretching exercises help fatigued muscles reestablish their normal resting length and prevent unnecessary pain.

Designing a Flexibility Program

To improve body flexibility, each major muscle group should be subjected to at least one stretching exercise. A complete set of exercises

Mode:	Static stretching or proprioceptive neuromuscular facilitation (PNF)
Intensity:	Stretch to the point of mild discomfort
Repetitions:	Repeat each exercise 4 to 5 times, and hold the final stretched position for 10 to 60 seconds
Frequency:	2 to 6 days per week

FIGURE 3.6 ❖ Flexibility development guidelines.

for developing muscular flexibility is presented in Appendix C. You may not be able to hold a final stretched position with some of these exercises (such as lateral head tilts and arm circles), but you should still perform the exercise through the joint's full range of motion. Depending on the number and the length of repetitions, a complete workout will last between 15 and 30 minutes.

PREVENTION AND REHABILITATION OF LOW-BACK PAIN

Few people make it through life without having low-back pain at some point. An estimated 75 million Americans currently suffer from chronic low-back pain each year. About 80% of the time, backache is preventable and is caused by some combination of: (a) physical inactivity, (b) poor postural habits and body mechanics, and (c) excessive body weight.

Lack of physical activity is the most common contributor to chronic low-back pain. Deterioration or weakening of the abdominal and gluteal muscles, along with tightening of the lower back (erector spine) muscles, brings about an unnatural forward tilt of the pelvis (see Figure 3.7). This tilt puts extra pressure on the spinal vertebrae, causing pain in the lower back. Accumulation of fat around the midsection of the body contributes to the forward tilt of the pelvis, which further aggravates the condition.

Low-back pain frequently is associated with faulty posture and improper body mechanics in all of life's daily activities, including sleeping, sitting, standing, walking, driving, working, and exercising. Incorrect posture and poor mechanics, as explained in Figure 3.8, increase strain not only on the lower back but on many other bones, joints, muscles, and ligaments as well.

The incidence and frequency of low-back pain can be reduced greatly by including some specific stretching and strengthening exercises in the regular fitness program. In many cases, back pain is present only with movement and physical activity. If back pain is severe and persists even at rest, the first step is to consult a physician,

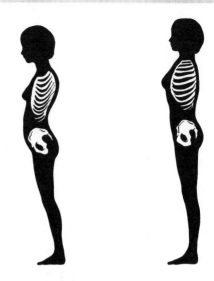

FIGURE 3.7 ❖ Incorrect (left) and correct (right) pelvic alignment.

who can rule out any disc damage and most likely will prescribe proper bed rest using several pillows under the knees for leg support (see Figure 3.8). This position helps release muscle spasms by stretching the muscles involved. In addition, a physician may prescribe a muscle relaxant or anti-inflammatory medication, or both, and some type of physical therapy.

Once the individual is pain-free in the resting state, he or she needs to start correcting the muscular imbalance by stretching the tight muscles and strengthening the weak ones. Stretching exercises are always done first.

Several exercises for preventing backache and rehabilitating the back are given in Appendix D. These exercises can be done twice or more daily when a person has back pain. Under normal circumstances, three to four times a week is sufficient to prevent the syndrome.

BIOMECHANICS OF EXERCISE

Biomechanics involves the study of the motion of humans and the effects that forces have on

HOW TO STAY ON YOUR FEET WITHOUT TIRING YOUR BACK

To prevent strain and pain in everyday activities, it is restful to change from one task to another before fatigue sets in. Housewives can lie down between chores; others should check body position frequently, drawing in the abdomen, flattening the back, bending the knees slightly.

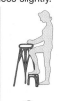

Not this way

Use of a footrest relieves swayback.

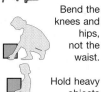

Not this way

Bend the knees and hips, not the waist.

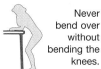

Not this way

Hold heavy objects close to you.

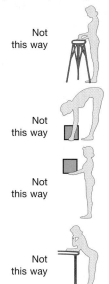

Not this way

Never bend over without bending the knees.

HOW TO PUT YOUR BACK TO BED

For proper bed posture, a firm mattress is essential. Bedboards, sold commercially, or devised at home, may be used with soft mattresses. Bedboards, preferably, should be made of 3/4 inch plywood. Faulty sleeping positions intensify swayback and result not only in backache but in numbness, tingling, and pain in arms and legs.

Incorrect:
Lying flat on back makes swayback worse.

Use of high pillow strains neck, arms, shoulders.

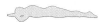

Sleeping face down exaggerates swayback, strains neck and shoulders.

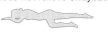

Bending one hip and knee does not relieve swayback.

Correct:
Lying on side with knees bent effectively flattens the back. Flat pillow may be used to support neck, especially when shoulders are broad.

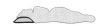

Sleeping on back is restful and correct when knees are properly supported.

Raise the foot of the mattress eight inches to discourage sleeping on the abdomen.

Proper arrangement of pillows for resting or reading in bed.

HOW TO SIT CORRECTLY

A back's best friend is a straight, hard chair. If you can't get the chair you prefer, learn to sit properly on whatever chair you get. To correct sitting position from forward slump: Throw head well back, then bend it forward to pull in the chin. This will straighten the back. Now tighten abdominal muscles to raise the chest. Check position frequently.

Relieve strain by sitting well forward, flatten back by tightening abdominal muscles, and cross knees.

Use of footrest relieves swayback. Aim is to have knees higher than hips.

Correct way to sit while driving, close to pedals. Use seatbelt or hard backrest, available commercially.

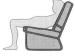

TV slump leads to "dowager's hump," strains neck and shoulders.

If chair is too high, swayback is increased.

Keep neck and back in as straight a line as possible with the spine. Bend forward from hips.

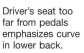

Driver's seat too far from pedals emphasizes curve in lower back.

Strained reading position. Forward thrusting strains muscles of neck and head.

FIGURE 3.8 ❖ Your back and how to care for it.

the body. As the number of individuals who participate in a regular exercise program has increased, so has the number of injuries associated with vigorous physical exercise. Expanded knowledge about the causes of injury aids in preventing many of these injuries.

Biomechanical analysis of exercise activities helps us to better understand how injuries occur. When vigorous activities are performed incorrectly, the forces acting on the body are greater, increasing the likelihood of injury. Performing activities in the most biomechanically efficient manner reduces the forces acting on the body and thus lessens the risk for injury. Therefore, participants would be wise to understand and use proper biomechanical technique during exercise.

Biomechanical Principles Related to Aerobic Activities

Aerobic activities such as walking, jogging, cycling, and aerobic dance involve repetitive movements that can place high demands on the musculoskeletal system. The following applications of biomechanical principles are related to four sample activities.

Walking

Walking has a very low risk for injury. The stresses imposed on the body are far less than those experienced in an activity such as running. During walking the individual should maintain a vertical posture and point the toes straight ahead. Excessive forward lean strains the back muscles, and toeing in or out can create stress at the knee and hip.

Walking speed is a function of stride length and stride rate. Most individuals naturally set a cadence that is comfortable and most efficient for them. Mechanical efficiency for most people is best when walking between 2.5 and 3.0 miles per hour (20 to 24 minutes per mile). Walking faster increases the heart rate but also increases the mechanical stress on the body.

Jogging

The vertical ground reaction force acting on the body while jogging is around 2.5 to 3 times a person's body weight. For a person who weighs 150 pounds, this force is about 400 pounds every time the foot strikes the ground. Some individuals create even larger forces because of poor running mechanics. Proper running technique helps reduce these forces and decreases the jogger's risk for injury.

An important factor when jogging is the footstrike. As in walking, the toes should be pointed straight ahead. The runner should land on the heel and roll forward to the ball of the foot. The knee should be bent during landing and then bend slightly more as the leg receives the body's weight. Proper foot and knee actions help dissipate the landing force.

A common fault among runners is to allow the toe to point outward at landing. When this happens, the landing force causes the foot to roll inward and flattens the arch. This action is called pronation. Although some pronation is needed to help absorb the landing force, excessive pronation creates torsion (twisting) in the lower leg, increasing stress on the ankle and knee.

Proper footwear is important for joggers. Good running shoes help absorb some of the impact force from landing. Some shoes are designed to help control over-pronation. If you have a tendency to over-pronate, you should choose a running shoe with good lateral stability. Salespersons at most reputable athletic shoe stores are knowledgeable about running shoes and can help you select the proper shoe.

Cycling

Individuals who are concerned about impact forces in jogging often choose cycling for their aerobic exercise. Cycling certainly is less stressful from the standpoint of impact, but it is not without its hazards. Bicycle propulsion results from the action of the hips, knees, and ankles. The greatest stress is felt at the knee joint. Saddle height has a strong influence on the forces acting on the knee. If the seat is too low, the knee is placed at great biomechanical disadvantage, creating an overload that may lead to injury. If the seat is too high, the rider has to stretch at the bottom of each pedal stroke. This causes back-and-forth rotation of the pelvis, eventually causing back pain.

Of great significance also is the overall geometry of the bicycle, which should fit your body's dimensions. If the bike is too large or too small, the body is placed in an uncomfortable position, which increases with increased riding time. If the body has to lean too far forward, the arms and back are required to support too much of the weight. The stress from this overload eventually causes injury. A bicycle salesperson can help select the bicycle that is right for you.

Biomechanical efficiency in cycling is attained with the proper combination of pedaling rate and the force applied to the pedal. The gears on a bicycle help you maintain this optimal level of efficiency. Most road bikes have ten or twelve gears. Mountain bikes generally have eighteen to twenty-one gears. Riding in low gears requires less force but a faster pedaling rate. The lower gears typically are used to climb hills. Riding in higher gears requires more force but lower pedaling rates. The greater the force applied to the pedal, the greater is the stress on the knees.

Because biomechanical efficiency is attained at the optimum combination of force and speed, too little speed hurts efficiency. Studies have found that efficiency in cycling is best when the pedaling rate is around 100 revolutions per minute (rpm). Many people tend to ride in too high a gear, which places excessive force on the knees. It is better to ride in a gear that requires you to apply less force to the pedals and allows you to pedal at 60 rpm or more.

Aerobics

High-impact aerobic dance (see Chapter 4) is often cited for its extremely high injury rate. The repetitive shock of landing creates forces similar to those in running. Consequently, problems and their solutions are similar to those for joggers. A large number of aerobic dance injuries occur from poor biomechanical control of the foot and leg. Proper vertical alignment of the feet, knees, and hips greatly alleviates, and often eliminates, heel pain, shin pain, knee pain, hip pain, and low back pain. Proper footwear also helps to avoid injury.

Because of the increased risk for injury associated with high-impact aerobics, most aerobic dance classes now employ low-impact routines. In low-impact aerobics the performer keeps one foot on the ground most of the time, eliminating the high-impact landings that result from the airborne phase associated with high-impact aerobics. Low-impact routines include more side-to-side movements rather than up-and-down movements. Injuries still occur in low-impact aerobics but not to the extent they do in high-impact aerobics.

Another form of aerobics that has grown in popularity in recent years is step aerobics. Step aerobics involves stepping up on and down from a bench between 2" and 10" high. Step aerobics can provide a cardiorespiratory workout equivalent to running at 7 mph but with only half the impact force acting on the body. With such low stress and high aerobic benefit, no wonder many have chosen step aerobics as their preferred form of aerobic exercise.

The area of the body most susceptible to injury during step aerobics is the knee. The higher the step, the greater is the stress on the knee. Also, the higher the bench, the greater is the landing force when the person steps down to the floor.

Of utmost importance is to choose the proper step height for the person's height, skill level, and fitness level. When stepping on a bench, steppers should have to flex the knee no more than 90°. Individuals with a history of knee problems should be discouraged from participating in step aerobics.

Proper stepping technique also lowers the risk for injury. This entails keeping the knees bent and the posture erect. Too much forward lean places excessive stress on the lower back. Place the entire foot onto the bench during each step-up. Upon return to the floor, land first on the ball of the foot, then bring the heel down to the floor.

Biomechanical Principles Related to Muscular Strength and Endurance

Several biomechanical factors affect the amount of force an individual is capable of producing. These factors have implications for strength training and should be understood before designing a strength-training program. Biomechanical factors that affect strength measures are (a) type of muscular contraction (isotonic and isometric), (b) position of body segments, and (c) speed of movement. Each of these factors is discussed next.

Type of Contraction

Muscles are capable of producing the most force during eccentric movements, such as when lowering a resistance. A person often can lower a resistance in a controlled manner even though he or she may not be strong enough to lift that same resistance. An important concept is that when lifting and lowering the resistance, the same muscles are working. When doing a pull-up, for example, the biceps perform much of the work — both in raising and in lowering the body. The biceps contract concentrically (shorten) as you pull up and eccentrically (lengthen) as the body is lowered.

Position of Body Segments

The position of the body segments greatly influences the ability to produce force. One biomechanical factor involved is the length-tension relationship. When a muscle is stretched, it can produce more force. As it shortens, it produces less and less force. A second factor influenced by joint position is the angle of muscle pull. As a segment moves through its range of motion (ROM), the angle of muscle pull changes. A muscle is most effective when pulling at an angle close to 90°. It is less effective when pulling at smaller angles. The end result of the interaction of these two biomechanical factors is that the muscle's ability to produce force varies through the segment's ROM.

Speed of Movement

The force a muscle can produce varies inversely with the speed at which the muscle is shortening. That is, force decreases as speed increases. For example, a shot putter must exert a large force to get the shot moving from its stationary position, but as the shot increases in speed, it becomes more difficult for the shot putter to continue to apply force to the shot.

Skill and Strength Training

Lifting weights is a skill just like any other; a learning process is involved. As you practice, your skill level will improve and you will become more efficient. At first your ability to lift an increasing amount of resistance is as much a result of improved skill as it is increased strength. For this reason, some fitness leaders recommend that you begin a strength-training program using light resistance and more repetitions. Once you have learned to lift weights safely and efficiently, you may begin to increase the resistance.

TIPS TO ENHANCE ADHERENCE TO EXERCISE

Starting and maintaining a fitness program is not easy if you are not accustomed to an exercise program. Introducing new behaviors into life's daily routine takes most people months to accomplish. A fitness program is no exception. Adding exercise to a person's lifestyle may require retraining (behavior modification).

Different things motivate different people to start and remain in a fitness program. Regardless of the initial reason for initiating an exercise program, you now need to plan for ways to make your workout fun. The psychology behind it is simple: If you enjoy an activity, you will continue to do it. If you don't, you will quit. Some of the following suggestions may help:

1. Start slowly. One of the most common mistakes people make with exercise is doing

too much too quickly. This increases the risk for injuries and often leads to discouragement and dropping out. Keep in mind that the body's conditioning process takes months.

2. Select aerobic activities you enjoy doing. Picking an activity you don't enjoy makes you less likely to keep exercising.

3. Combine various activities. Train by doing two or three different activities the same week. This makes exercising less monotonous than repeating the same activity again and again.

4. Find a friend or group of friends to exercise with. Social interaction will make exercise more fulfilling. Besides, it's harder to skip if someone is waiting for you.

5. Set aside a regular time for exercise. If you don't plan ahead, it's a lot easier to skip. Holding your exercise hour "sacred" will help you adhere to the program.

6. Obtain the proper equipment for exercise. A poor pair of shoes, for instance, can increase the risk for injury, discouraging you right from the beginning.

7. Don't become a chronic exerciser. Learn to listen to our body. Overexercising can lead to chronic fatigue and injuries. Exercise should be enjoyable, and in the process you will need to "stop and smell the roses."

8. Exercise in different places and facilities to add variety to your workouts.

9. Conduct periodic assessments. Improving to a higher fitness category is a reward in itself.

10. Keep a regular record of your activities. This allows you to monitor your progress and compare it with previous months and years. Use forms similar to those in Figures 3.10 and 3.11 to monitor your aerobic and strength-training programs.

11. See a physician if health problems arise. When in doubt, it's "better safe than sorry."

12. Set goals and share them with others. Quitting is tougher when someone knows what you are trying to accomplish. When you reach a specific goal, reward yourself with a new pair of shoes or a jogging suit.

SETTING FITNESS GOALS

Before you leave this chapter, you must consider your fitness goals. In the last few decades we have become accustomed to "quick fixes" with everything from super fast foods to one-hour dry cleaning. Fitness, however, has no quick fix. Fitness takes time and dedication to develop, and only those who are committed and persistent will reap the rewards. As described in Chapter 1, setting realistic fitness goals will help you design and guide your program. Figure 3.9 offers a goal-setting chart that will help you determine your fitness goals. Take the time, either by yourself or with your instructor's help, to fill it out.

As you prepare to write realistic fitness goals, base these goals on the results of your initial fitness test (pre-test). For instance, if your cardiorespiratory fitness category was poor on the pre-test, you should not expect to improve to the excellent category in a little more than 3 months.

Whenever possible, your fitness goals should be measurable. A goal that simply states "to improve cardiorespiratory endurance" is not as measurable as a goal that states "to improve to the good fitness category in cardiorespiratory endurance" or "to run the 1.5–mile course in less than 11 minutes."

After determining each goal, you also will need to write measurable objectives to accomplish that goal. These objectives will be the actual plan of action to accomplish your goal. A sample of objectives to accomplish the previously stated goal for cardiorespiratory endurance development could be:

1. Use jogging as the mode of exercise.

2. Jog at 10:00 a.m. five times per week.

3. Jog around the track in the fieldhouse.

4. Jog for 30 minutes each exercise session.

5. Monitor heart rate regularly during exercise.
6. Take the 1.5-Mile Run Test once a month.

Specific objectives will not always be met. Consequently, your goal may be out of reach. If so, reevaluate your objectives and make adjustments accordingly. If you set unrealistic goals at the beginning of your exercise program, be flexible with yourself and reconsider your plan of action but do not quit. Reconsidering your plan of action does not mean failure. Failure comes only to those who stop trying, and success comes to those who are committed and persistent.

NOTES

1. American College of Sports Medicine, *Guidelines for Exercise Testing and Prescription* (Baltimore: Williams & Wilkins, 1995).
2. R. F. DeBusk, U. Stenestrand, M. Sheehan, and W. L. Haskell, "Training Effects of Long Versus Short Bouts of Exercise in Healthy Subjects," *American Journal of Cardiology*, 65 (1990), 1010–1013.
3. U. S. Centers for Disease Control and Prevention and American College of Sports Medicine, "Summary Statement: Workshop on Physical Activity and Public Health," *Sports Medicine Bulletin*, 28:4 (1993), 7.
4. American College of Sports Medicine, "The Recommended Quantity and Quality of Exercise for Developing and Maintaining Cardiorespiratory and Muscular Fitness in Healthy Adults," *Medicine and Science in Sports and Exercise*, 22 (1990), 265–274.
5. J. Kokkonen and S. Lauritzen, "Isotonic Strength and Endurance Gains Through PNF Stretching," *Medicine and Science in Sports and Exercise*, 27 (1995), S22:127.

Indicate below two or three general goals that you will work on during the next few weeks, and write the specific objectives you will use to accomplish each goal.

Cardiorespiratory endurance goal: _____

_____

Specific objectives:

1._____

2._____

3._____

4._____

5._____

6._____

_____   _____
My signature   Witness signature

_____   _____
Today's date   Date of completion

Muscular strength/endurance goal: _____

_____

Specific objectives:

1._____

2._____

3._____

4._____

5._____

6._____

_____   _____
My signature   Witness signature

_____   _____
Today's date   Date of completion

FIGURE 3.9 ❖ Goal-setting chart.

Muscular flexibility goal:_____

_____

Specific objectives:

1._____

2._____

3._____

4._____

5._____

6._____

_____   _____
My signature   Witness signature

_____   _____
Today's date   Date of completion

Body composition goal: _____

_____

Specific objectives:

1._____

2._____

3._____

4._____

5._____

6._____

_____   _____
My signature   Witness signature

_____   _____
Today's date   Date of completion

FIGURE 3.9 ❖ Goal-setting chart (continued).

Aerobics Record Form

Date	Body Weight	Exercise Heart Rate	Type of Exercise	Distance in Miles	Time Hrs./Min.
1					
2					
3					
4					
5					
6					
7					
8					
9					
10					
11					
12					
13					
14					
15					
16					
17					
18					
19					
20					
21					
22					
23					
24					
25					
26					
27					
28					
29					
30					
31					
			Total		

FIGURE 3.10 ❖ Aerobics record form (make additional copies as needed).

Strength Training Record Form

Name _____

Date _____

Exercise	St/Reps/Res*	St/Reps/Res*	St/Reps/Res*	St/Reps/Res*	St/Reps/Res*	St/Reps/Res*	St/Reps/Res*	St/Reps/Res*	St/Reps/Res*	St/Reps/Res*

* St/Reps/Res = Sets, Repetitions, and Resistance (e.g., 1/6/125 = 1 set of 6 repetitions with 125 pounds)

FIGURE 3.11 ❖ Strength training record form (make additional copies as needed).

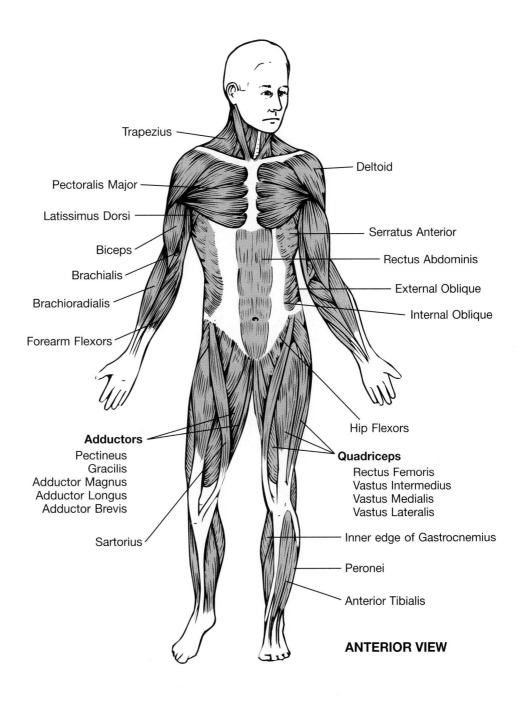

Trapezius

Deltoid

Pectoralis Major

Latissimus Dorsi

Serratus Anterior

Biceps

Rectus Abdominis

Brachialis

External Oblique

Brachioradialis

Internal Oblique

Forearm Flexors

Hip Flexors

Adductors
Pectineus
Gracilis
Adductor Magnus
Adductor Longus
Adductor Brevis

Quadriceps
Rectus Femoris
Vastus Intermedius
Vastus Medialis
Vastus Lateralis

Inner edge of Gastrocnemius

Peronei

Sartorius

Anterior Tibialis

ANTERIOR VIEW

FIGURE 3.12 ❖ Major muscles of the human body.

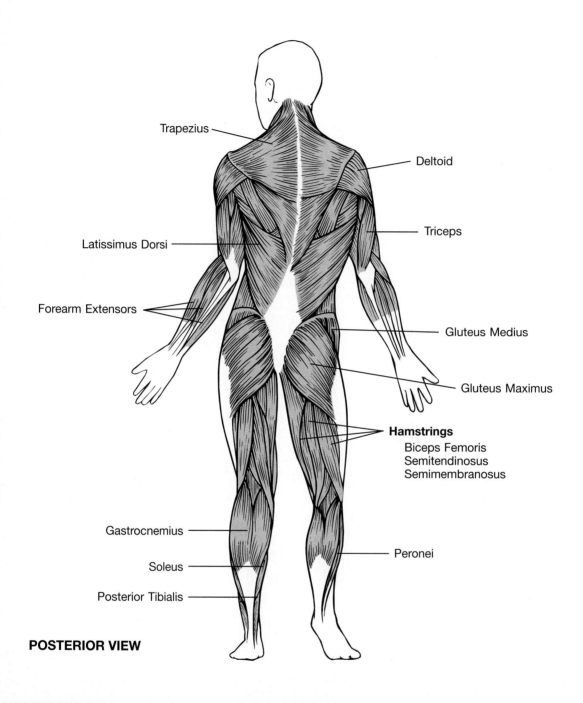

Trapezius

Deltoid

Latissimus Dorsi

Triceps

Forearm Extensors

Gluteus Medius

Gluteus Maximus

Hamstrings
Biceps Femoris
Semitendinosus
Semimembranosus

Gastrocnemius

Peronei

Soleus

Posterior Tibialis

POSTERIOR VIEW

FIGURE 3.12 ❖ Major muscles of the human body (continued).

Evaluating Fitness Activities

KEY TERMS

Aero-belt exercise

Aerobic dance (aerobics)

Aerobic-fitness

Cross-training

High-impact aerobics (HIA)

Low-impact aerobics (LIA)

MET (metabolic equivalent)

~~Sk~~...

~~Step~~ aerobics (SA)

OBJECTIVES

✤ Learn the benefits and advantages of selected aerobic activities.

✤ Learn to rate the fitness benefits of aerobic activities.

✤ Evaluate the contributions of skill-related fitness activities.

✤ Understand the sequence of a standard aerobic workout.

✤ Learn ways to enhance aerobic workouts.

...es of exercise is that many different activities promoting fitness are available from which to choose. You may select one or a combination of activities for your program. The choice should be based on personal enjoyment, convenience, and availability.

AEROBIC ACTIVITIES

Most people who exercise pick and adhere to a single mode, such as walking, swimming, or jogging. No single activity develops total fitness. Many activities contribute to cardiorespiratory development. The extent of contribution to other fitness components is limited, though, and varies among the activities. For total fitness, aerobic activities should be supplemented with strength and flexibility exercises. Selecting a combination of aerobic activities, cross-training, can add enjoyment to the program, decrease the risk of injuries from overuse, and keep exercise from becoming monotonous.

Exercise sessions should be convenient. To enjoy exercise, a time should be selected when you will not be rushed. A nearby location is recommended. People do not enjoy driving across town to get to the gym, health club, track, or pool. If parking is a problem, you may get discouraged quickly and quit. All these factors are used as excuses not to stick to an exercise program.

Walking

The most natural, easiest, safest, and least expensive form of aerobic exercise is walking. For years, many fitness practitioners believed that walking was not vigorous enough to improve cardiorespiratory functioning. Now studies have established that brisk walking at speeds of 4 miles per hour or faster improves cardiorespiratory fitness. From a health-fitness viewpoint, a regular walking program can prolong life

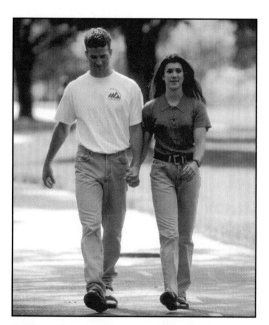

Walking, the most natural aerobic exercise.

significantly (see the discussion of cardiovascular disease in Chapter 7). Although walking takes longer than jogging, the caloric cost of brisk walking is only about 10% lower than jogging the same distance.

Walking is perhaps the best activity to start a conditioning program for the cardiorespiratory system. Inactive people should start with 1-mile walks four to five times per week. Walk times can be increased gradually by 5 minutes each week. Following 3 to 4 weeks of conditioning, people should be able to walk 2 miles at a 4-mile-per-hour pace, five times per week. For greater aerobic benefits, walk longer and swing the arms faster than normal. Light hand weights, a backpack (4 to 6 pounds), or an Aero-belt (discussed later in this chapter) also add to the intensity of walking. Because of the additional load on the cardiorespiratory system, extra weights or loads are not recommended for people who have cardiovascular disease.

Walking in water (chest-deep level) is an excellent form of activity for people with leg and back problems. Because of the buoyancy that water provides, individuals submerged in water to armpit level weigh only about 10% to 20% of their weight outside the water. The resistance the water creates as a person walks in the pool makes the intensity quite high, providing an excellent cardiorespiratory workout.

Hiking

Hiking is an excellent activity for the entire family, especially during the summer and on summer vacations. Many people feel guilty if they are unable to continue their exercise routine during vacations. The intensity of hiking over uneven terrain is greater than walking. An 8-hour hike can burn as many calories as a 20-mile walk or jog.

Another benefit of hiking is the relaxing effects of beautiful scenery. This is an ideal activity for highly stressed people who live near woods and hills. A rough day at the office can be forgotten quickly in the peacefulness and beauty of the outdoors.

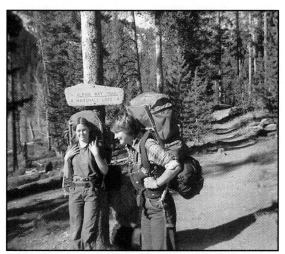

An 8-hour hike can burn as many calories as a 20-mile walk or jog.

Jogging/Running

Jogging is the most popular form of aerobic exercise. Next to walking, it is one of the most accessible forms of exercise. A person can find places to jog almost everywhere. The lone requirement to prevent injuries is a good pair of jogging shoes.

The popularity of jogging in the United States started shortly after publication of Dr. Kenneth Cooper's first aerobics book in 1968. Jim Fixx's *Complete Book of Running* in the mid 1970s further contributed to the phenomenal growth of jogging as the predominant fitness activity in the United States.

Jogging three to five times a week is one of the fastest ways to improve cardiorespiratory fitness. The risk of injury, however, especially among beginners, is greater with jogging than walking. For proper conditioning, jogging programs should start with 1 to 2 weeks of walking. As fitness improves, walking and jogging can be combined, gradually increasing the jogging segment until it comprises the full 20 to 30 minutes.

Many people abuse this activity. People run too fast and too long. Some joggers think that if a little is good, more is better. Not so with cardiorespiratory endurance. As indicated under "Frequency of Exercise" in Chapter 3, the aerobic benefits of training more than 30 minutes five times per week are minimal. Furthermore, the risk of injury increases greatly as speed (running instead of jogging) and mileage go up. Jogging approximately 15 miles per week is sufficient to reach an excellent level of cardiorespiratory fitness.

A good pair of shoes is a must for joggers. Many foot, knee, and leg problems originate from improperly fitting or worn-out shoes. A good pair of shoes should offer good lateral stability and not lean to either side when placed on a flat surface. The shoe also should bend at the ball of the foot, not at midfoot. Worn-out shoes should be replaced. After 500 miles of use, jogging shoes lose about a third of their shock absorption capabilities. If you suddenly have problems, check your shoes first. It may be time for a new pair.

For safety reasons, joggers should stay away from high-speed roads, not wear headphones, and always run (or walk) against the traffic so they will be able to see all oncoming traffic. At night, reflective clothing or fluorescent material should be worn on different parts of the body. Carrying a flashlight is even better because motorists can see the light from a greater distance than the reflective material.

An alternative form of jogging, especially for injured people, those with chronic back problems, and overweight individuals, is deep-water running (running in place while treading water). Deep-water running is almost as strenuous as jogging on land. In deep-water running, the running motions used on land are accentuated by pumping the arms and legs hard through a full range of motion. The participant usually wears a floatation vest to help maintain the body in an upright position. Many elite athletes train frequently in water to lessen the wear and tear on the body caused by long-distance running. These athletes have been able to maintain high oxygen uptake values through rigorous water running programs.

Aerobics

Aerobics, formerly known as aerobic dance, is thought to be the most common fitness activity for women in the United States. Aerobics involves *a series of exercise routines performed to music*. Routines consist of a combination of stepping, walking, jogging, skipping, kicking, and arm-swinging movements. It is a fun way to exercise and promote cardiorespiratory development at the same time.

Aerobics was developed initially in the early 1970s by Jacki Sorenson as a fitness program for Air Force wives in Puerto Rico. At first considered a fad, it now is a legitimate fitness activity with more than 20 million participants of all ages. Aerobics now are part of school curricula, health clubs, and recreational facilities.

High-impact aerobics (HIA), the traditional form of aerobics, involves *actions in which both feet may be off the floor momentarily at the same time*. These movements exert a great amount of vertical force on the feet as they contact the floor. Proper leg conditioning through other forms of weight-bearing aerobic exercises (brisk walking and jogging), as well as strength training, are recommended prior to participation in high-impact aerobics.

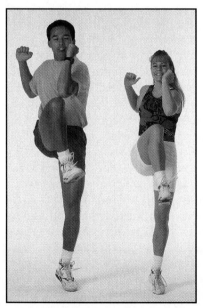

Aerobics, the most popular fitness activity for women in the United States.

High-impact aerobics is an intense activity, and it also produces the highest rate of aerobics injuries. Shin splints, stress fractures, low-back pain, and tendinitis are all too common in high-impact aerobics enthusiasts. These injuries are caused by the constant impact of the feet on firm surfaces. As a result, several alternative forms of aerobics have been developed.

Low-impact aerobics (LIA) require *movements in which at least one foot is in contact with the floor or ground at all times*, reducing the impact as each foot contacts the surface. The recommended exercise intensity is more difficult to maintain with low-impact aerobics, though. To help elevate the exercise heart rate, all arm movements and weight-bearing actions that lower the center of gravity should be accentuated. Sustained movement throughout the program is also crucial to keep the heart rate in the target cardiorespiratory zone.

A relatively new form of aerobics is step aerobics (SA). Using *a combination of stepping and arm movements*, participants step up and down benches that range in height from 2 to 10 inches. Step aerobics adds another dimension to the aerobics movement and an exercise program. As noted previously, variety adds enjoyment to aerobic workouts.

Step aerobics is viewed as a high-intensity but low-impact activity. The intensity of the activity can be controlled easily by the height of the steps. Aerobic benches or plates are now commercially available. These plates can be stacked together safely to adjust the height of the steps. Beginners are encouraged to use the lowest stepping height and then advance gradually to a higher bench. This practice will decrease the risk for injury. Even though one foot is always in contact with the floor or bench during step aerobics, this activity is not recommended for individuals with ankle, knee, or hip problems.

Other forms of aerobics include a combination of HIA and LIA, as well as moderate-impact aerobics (MIA). The latter incorporates plyometric training. Plyometric aerobics requires *forceful jumps or springing off the ground immediately after landing from a previous jump.* This type of training is used frequently by jumpers (high, long, and triple jumpers) and athletes in sports that require quick jumping ability, such as basketball and gymnastics.

With moderate-impact aerobics, one foot is in contact with the ground most of the time. Participants, however, continually try to recover from all lower-body flexion actions. This is done by extending the hip, knee, and ankle joints quickly without allowing the foot (or feet) to leave the ground. These quick movements make the exercise intensity of moderate-impact aerobics quite high.

Swimming

Swimming is another excellent form of aerobic exercise. It uses almost all major muscle groups in the body, providing a good training stimulus for the heart and lungs. Swimming is a great exercise option for individuals who cannot jog or walk for extended periods.

Compared to other activities, the risk of injuries from swimming is low. The aquatic medium helps to support the body, taking pressure off bones and joints in the lower extremities and the back.

Maximal heart rates during swimming are approximately 10 to 13 beats per minute (bpm) lower than during running.[1] The horizontal position of the body is thought to aid blood flow distribution throughout the body, decreasing the demand on the cardiorespiratory system. Cool water temperatures and direct contact with the water seem to help dissipate body heat more efficiently, further decreasing the strain on the heart.

Some exercise specialists recommend that this difference in maximal heart rate (10 to 13 bpm) be subtracted prior to determining cardiorespiratory training intensities. For example, the estimated maximal swimming heart rate for a 20-year old would be approximately 187 bpm (220 − 20 − 13).

Studies are inconclusive as to whether this decrease in heart rate in water also occurs at submaximal intensities below 70% of maximal

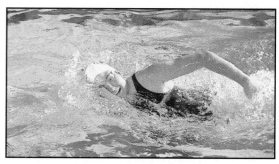
Swimming, a relatively injury-free activity.

heart rate.[2,3,4] Further, research comparing physiologic differences between self-paced treadmill running and self-paced water aerobics exercise showed that individuals work at lower intensities in water.[5] One can argue, therefore, that apparently healthy people are able to achieve higher work capacities during land-based activities; therefore, the same exercise intensity can be given for water activities. If a lower intensity is used, training benefits may be decreased.

To produce better training benefits during swimming, gliding periods such as those in the breast stroke and side stroke should be minimized. Achieving proper training intensities with these strokes is difficult. The forward crawl is recommended for better aerobic results.

Overweight individuals need to swim fast enough to achieve an adequate training intensity. Excessive body fat makes the body more buoyant, and often the tendency is to just float along. This may be good for reducing stress and relaxing, but it does not increase caloric expenditure to aid with weight loss. Walking or jogging in waist- or armpit-deep water are better choices for overweight individuals who cannot walk or jog on land for a long time.

With reference to the principle of specificity of training, swimming participants need to realize that cardiorespiratory improvements cannot be measured adequately with a walk/jog test. Most of the work with swimming is done by the upper body musculature. Although the heart's ability to pump a greater amount of oxygenated blood improves significantly with any type of aerobic activity, the primary increase in the ability of cells to utilize oxygen (VO_2 or oxygen uptake) with swimming occurs in the upper body and not the lower extremities. Therefore, fitness improvements with swimming are best attained by comparing changes in distances a person swims in a given time, say, 10 minutes.

Water Aerobics

This relatively new form of exercise is fun and safe for people of all ages. Besides developing fitness, water aerobics provides an opportunity for socialization and fun in a comfortable and refreshing setting.

Water aerobics incorporates a combination of rhythmic arm and leg actions performed in a vertical position while submerged in waist- to armpit-deep water. The vigorous limb movements against the water's resistance during water aerobics provide the training stimuli for cardiorespiratory development.

The popularity of water aerobics as an exercise modality to develop the cardiorespiratory system has been on the rise in recent years. This increase in popularity can be attributed to several factors:

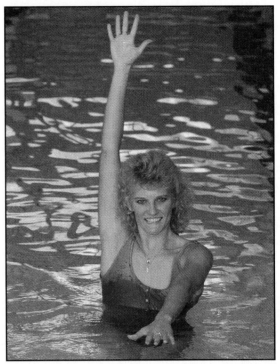

Water aerobics, fitness, fun, and safety for people of all ages.

1. Water buoyancy reduces weight-bearing stress on joints and therefore lessens the risk for injuries.
2. Water aerobics is a more feasible type of exercise for overweight individuals and those with arthritic conditions who may not be able to participate in weight-bearing activities such as walking, jogging, and aerobics.
3. Heat dissipation in water is beneficial to obese participants who seem to undergo a higher heat strain than average-weight individuals.
4. Water aerobics is available to swimmers and nonswimmers alike.

The exercises used during water aerobics are designed to elevate the heart rate, which contributes to cardiorespiratory development. In addition, the aquatic medium provides increased resistance for strength improvement with virtually no impact. Because of this resistance to movement, strength gains with water aerobics seem to be better than with other land-based aerobic activities. Water exercises also help the joints move through their range of motion, promoting flexibility.

Another benefit is that weight reduction can be facilitated without pain and fear of injuries experienced by many who initiate exercise programs. Water aerobics provides a relatively safe environment for injury-free participation in exercise. The cushioned environment of the water allows patients recovering from leg and back injuries, individuals with joint problems, injured athletes, pregnant women, and obese people to benefit from water aerobics. In water, these people can exercise to develop and maintain cardiorespiratory endurance and yet limit or eliminate the potential for further injury.

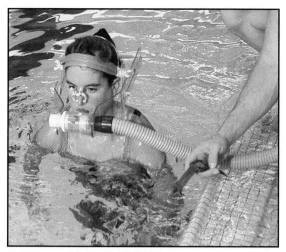
Oxygen uptake (VO$_2$) and heart rate assessment during water aerobics.

Similar to swimming, maximal heart rates achieved during water aerobics are lower than during running. The difference between water aerobics and running is about 10 bpm.[6] Apparently healthy people, nonetheless, can sustain land-based exercise intensities during a water aerobics workout and experience similar or greater fitness benefits than during land aerobics.[7] As with swimming, land-based exercise intensities, therefore, are recommended for water aerobics.

Cycling

Cycling is an activity that most people learn in their youth. As a non-weight-bearing activity, it is a good exercise modality for people with lower-body or lower-back injuries. Cycling helps to develop the cardiorespiratory system, as well as muscular strength and endurance in the lower extremities. With the advent of stationary bicycles, this activity can be performed year-round.

Raising the heart rate to the proper training intensity is more difficult with cycling. As the amount of muscle mass involved during aerobic exercise decreases, so does the demand placed on the cardiorespiratory system. The thigh muscles do most of the work in cycling, making it harder to achieve and maintain a high cardiorespiratory training intensity.

Maintaining a continuous pedaling motion and eliminating coasting periods helps the participant achieve a faster heart rate. Exercising for longer periods also helps to compensate for the lower heart rate intensity during cycling. When comparing cycling to jogging, similar aerobic benefits take roughly three times the distance at twice the speed of jogging. Cycling, however, puts less stress on muscles and joints than jogging does, making the former a better exercise modality for people who cannot otherwise walk or jog.

To increase riding efficiency, the height of the bike seat should be adjusted so the legs are almost completely extended when the heels are placed on the pedals. The body should not sway from side to side as the person rides. The cycling cadence also is important for maximal efficiency. Bike tension or gears should be set at a moderate level to be able to ride at 60 to 100 revolutions per minute.

Skill is important in road cycling. Cyclists must be in control of the bicycle at all times. They have to be able to maneuver the bike in

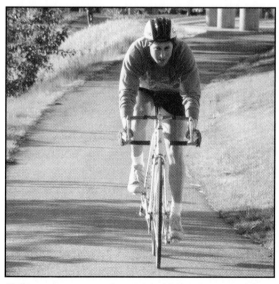
Skill is an important factor for safety and enjoyment of road cycling.

traffic, maintain balance at slow speeds, switch gears, apply the brakes, watch for pedestrians and stoplights, and ride through congested areas. Stationary cycling does not require special skills. Nearly everyone can do it.

Safety is a key issue in road cycling. More than a million bicycle injuries occur each year. Proper equipment and common sense are necessary. A well-designed and maintained bike is easier to maneuver. Toe clips are recommended to keep feet from sliding and to maintain equal upward and downward force on the pedals.

Bike riders must follow the same rules as motorists. Many accidents happen because cyclists run traffic lights and stop signs. Some further suggestions are:

❖ Use bike hand signals to let the traffic around you know of your actions.

❖ Don't ride side by side with another rider.

❖ Be aware of turning vehicles and cars backing out of alleys and parking lots; always yield to motorists in these situations.

❖ Avoid storm drains, which can cause unpleasant surprises; if you do not cross them at the proper angle, front wheels can get caught and riders may be thrown from the bike.

❖ Wear a good helmet, certified by the Snell Memorial Foundation or the American National Standards Institute. Many serious accidents and even deaths have been prevented by adequate use of helmets. Fashion, aesthetics, comfort, or price should not be a factor when selecting and using a helmet for road cycling. Health and life are too precious to give up because of vanity and thriftiness.

❖ Wear appropriate clothes and shoes. Special clothing for cycling is not required. Clothing should be lightweight and not restrict movement. Shorts should be long enough to keep the skin from rubbing against the seat. For greater comfort, cycling shorts have extra padding sewn into the seat and crotch areas. Experienced cyclists often wear special shoes with a cleat that snaps directly onto the pedal.

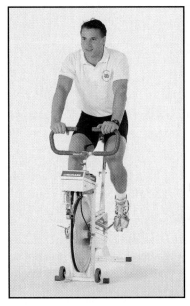

Exercising on a stationary bicycle adds variety to aerobic workouts.

The stationary bike is the most popular piece of equipment sold by sporting good stores. Before buying a stationary bike, though, be sure to try the activity for a few days. If you enjoy it, you may want to purchase one. Invest with caution. If you opt to buy a lower-priced model, you may be disappointed. Good stationary bikes have comfortable seats, are stable, and provide a smooth and uniform pedaling motion. A sticky bike that is hard to pedal only leads to discouragement and ends up stored in the corner of a basement.

Aero-Belt Exercise

A new mode of aerobic activity is Aero-belt exercise. The Aero-belt™ (Aerobic Endurance Resistance Overloader) consists of a belt with an elastic band that slides freely through the belt and attaches to the wrists.* The objective of using the Aero-belt is to provide resistance to the arms during lower body physical activity, thereby increasing the person's oxygen con-

---

*Aero-belt is a registered trademark of Nurge Fitness Systems, P.O. Box 889, Ketchum, ID 83340 Phone 1–800–879–8695.

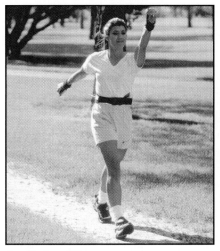

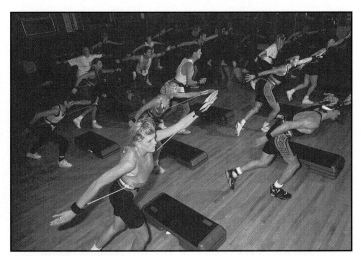

Aero-belt walking.　　　　　　　　　*Aero-belt step-aerobics.*

sumption, energy expenditure, and development of upper-body strength and endurance during aerobic exercise. As in cross-country skiing, the Aero-belt provides resistance to the arms while walking, jogging, bounding, stair stepping, riding a stationary bicycle, or doing aerobics.

Using the Aero-belt actually can provide more upper-body conditioning benefits than cross-country skiing. Three different tension grades for the elastic cord are available for individual strength and fitness levels. Medium and high tension are mainly for strength conditioning, and low tension is for developing endurance.

The physiologic responses to Aero-belt walking (4.0 and 4.2 mph), jogging (6.0 mph) and step aerobics were investigated at Boise State University.[8,9,10] Increases in heart rate, oxygen uptake, and caloric expenditure ranged from 32% to 54% from regular walking, jogging, and step-aerobics to walking, jogging, and step-aerobics with an Aero-belt (see Figure 4.1).

Cross-Training

Cross-training combines two or more activities. This type of training is designed to enhance fitness, provide needed rest to tired muscles, decrease injuries, and eliminate the monotony and burnout of single-activity programs. Cross-training may combine aerobic and nonaerobic activities such as moderate jogging, speed training, and strength training.

Cross-training can produce better workouts than a single activity. For example, jogging develops the lower body and swimming builds the upper body. Rowing contributes to upper-body development and cycling builds the legs. Combining activities such as these provides good overall conditioning and at the same time helps to improve or maintain fitness. Cross-training also offers an opportunity to develop skill and have fun with different activities.

Speed training often is coupled with cross-training. Faster performance times in aerobic activities (running, cycling) are generated with speed or interval training. People who want to improve their running times often run shorter intervals at faster speeds than the actual racing pace. For example, a person wanting to run a 6-minute mile may run four 440-yard intervals at a speed of 1 minute and 20 seconds per interval. A 440-yard walk/jog can become a recovery interval between fast runs.

Strength training is used commonly with cross-training. Strength training helps to condition muscles, tendons, and ligaments. In many

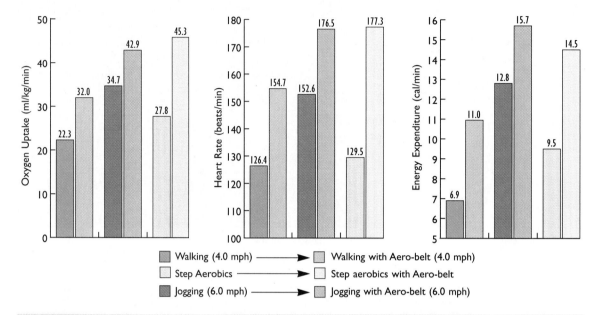

FIGURE 4.1 ❖ Oxygen uptake, heart rate, and energy expenditure responses to walking, jogging, and step aerobics with and without an Aero-belt.

activities improved strength enhances overall sports performance. For example, research has shown that although road cyclists who trained with weights showed no improvement in aerobic capacity, the cyclists had a 33% improvement in riding time to exhaustion when exercising at 75% of their maximal capacity.[11]

Rope Skipping

Rope skipping not only contributes to cardio-respiratory fitness, but it also helps to increase reaction time, coordination, agility, dynamic balance, and muscular strength in the lower extremities. At first rope skipping may appear to be a highly strenuous form of aerobic exercise. Beginners often reach maximal heart rates after only 2 or 3 minutes of jumping. As skill improves, however, the energy demands decrease considerably.

Some people have claimed training benefits equal to a 30-minute jog in as little as 10 minutes of skipping. Although differences in strength and flexibility development are observed in different activities, 10 minutes at a certain heart rate provide similar cardiorespiratory benefits regardless of the nature of the activity. To obtain an adequate aerobic workout, the duration of exercise must be at least 20 minutes.

As with high-impact aerobics, a major concern of rope skipping is the stress placed on the lower extremities. Skipping with one foot at a time decreases the impact somewhat, but it does not eliminate the risk for injuries. Fitness experts recommend that skipping be used sparingly and primarily as a supplement to an aerobic exercise program.

Cross-Country Skiing

Many consider cross-country skiing as the ultimate aerobic exercise because it requires vigorous lower and upper body movements. The large amount of muscle mass involved in cross-country skiing makes the intensity of the activity high, yet it places little strain on muscles and joints. One of the highest maximal oxygen uptakes ever measured (85 ml/kg/min) was found in an elite cross-country skier.

In addition to being an excellent aerobic activity, cross-country skiing is soothing. Skiing through the beauty of the snow-covered countryside can be highly enjoyable. Although the need for snow is an obvious limitation, cross-country skiing simulating equipment for year-round training is available at many sporting goods stores.

Some skill is necessary for proficient cross-country skiing. Poorly skilled individuals are not able to elevate the heart rate enough to cause adequate aerobic development. Individuals contemplating this activity should seek out instruction to fully enjoy and reap the rewards of cross-country skiing.

In-Line Skating

Frequently referred to as blading, in-line skating has become a highly popular fitness activity in recent years. Suddenly millions of children and adults are trying this activity. In the early 1990s stores could not keep up with the demand for in-line skates.

In-line skating has its origin in ice skating. Because warm-weather ice skating was not feasible, blades were replaced by wheels for summertime participation. Four-wheel roller skates were invented in the mid 1700s, but the activity did not really catch on until the late 1800s. The first in-line skate with five wheels in a row attached to the bottom of a shoe was developed in 1823. The in-line concept took hold in the United States in 1980, when hockey skates were adapted for this road-skating.

In-line skating is an excellent activity to develop cardiorespiratory fitness and lower body strength. The intensity of the activity is regulated by how hard you blade. The key to effective cardiorespiratory training is to maintain a constant and rhythmic pattern, using arms and legs, and minimizing the gliding phase of blading. As a weight-bearing activity, in-line bladers also develop superior leg strength.

Instruction is necessary to achieve a minimum level of proficiency in this sport. Bladers commonly encounter hazards. Potholes, cracks, rocks, gravel, sticks, oil, street curbs, and driveways all pose challenges. Unskilled bladers are more prone to falls and injuries.

Good equipment will make the activity safer and more enjoyable. Blades range in price from $40 to $500. Recreational participants need not purchase the more costly competitive skates. An adequate blade should provide strong ankle support. Soft and flexible boots do not provide enough support. Small wheels offer more stability, and larger wheels enable greater speed. Blades should be purchased from stores that understand the sport and can provide sound advice according to skill level and needs.

Protective equipment is a must for in-line skating. Similar to road cycling, a good helmet that meets the safety standards set by the Snell Memorial Foundation or the American Standards Institute is important to protect yourself in case of a fall. Wrist guards and knee and elbow pads also are recommended. The kneecap and the elbows are easily injured in any fall. Nighttime bladers should wear light-colored clothing and reflective tape.

Rowing

Rowing is a low-impact activity that provides a complete body workout. It mobilizes the use of most major muscle groups including the arms, legs, hips, abdominals, trunk, and shoulders. Rowing not only is a good form of aerobic exercise but, because of the nature of the activity (constant pushing and pulling against resistance), also promotes total strength development.

To accommodate different fitness levels, workloads can be regulated on most rowing machines. Rowing, however, is not among the most popular forms of aerobic exercise. Similar to stationary bicycles, people should try the activity for a few weeks before purchasing a unit.

Stair Climbing

If sustained for at least 20 minutes, stair climbing is an extremely efficient form of aerobic exercise. Precisely because of the high intensity of stair climbing, many people in our society stay away from stairs and instead ride elevators! Many people dislike living in two-story homes because they have to climb the stairs frequently.

Not too many places have enough flights of stairs to climb continuously for 20 minutes. Stair-climbing machines offer an alternative. Stair climbing has become so popular that fitness enthusiasts often wait in line at health clubs to use the machines.

In terms of injuries, stair climbing seems to be a relatively safe exercise modality. Because the feet never leave the climbing surface, it is considered a low-impact activity. Joints and ligaments are not really strained during climbing. The intensity of exercise is controlled easily because most stair climbers can be programmed to regulate the workload.

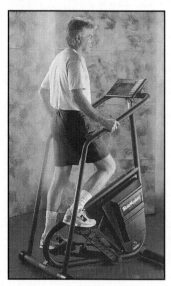

Stair climbing provides a rigorous aerobic workout.

Racquet Sports

In racquet sports such as tennis, racquetball, squash, and badminton, the aerobic benefits are dictated by players' skill, intensity of the game, and how long they play the game. Skill is

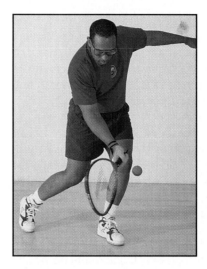

Racquet sports require rhythmic and continuous activity to provide aerobic benefits.

necessary not only to participate effectively in these sports but also is crucial to sustain continuous play. Frequent pauses during play do not allow people to maintain the heart rate in the appropriate target zone to stimulate cardiorespiratory development.

Many people who participate in racquet sports do so for enjoyment, social fulfillment, and relaxation. For cardiorespiratory fitness development these people supplement the sport with other forms of aerobic exercise such as jogging, cycling, or swimming.

If a racquet sport is the main form of aerobic exercise, participants need to try to run hard, fast, and as constantly as possible during play. They should not have to spend much time retrieving balls (bird or shuttlecock in badminton). Similar to low-impact aerobics, all movements should be accentuated by reaching out and bending more than usual, for better cardiorespiratory development.

RATING THE FITNESS BENEFITS OF AEROBIC ACTIVITIES

The fitness contributions of the aerobic activities discussed in this chapter vary according to activities and individuals. As noted previously, the health-related components of physical fitness are cardiorespiratory endurance, muscular strength and endurance, muscular flexibility, and body composition. Although an accurate assessment of the contributions to each fitness component are difficult to establish, a summary of likely benefits of these activities is provided in Table 4.1. Instead of a single rating or number, ranges are given for some of the categories. This is done because the benefits derived are based on the person's effort while participating in the activity.

Regular participation in aerobic activities provides notable health benefits, including an increase in cardiorespiratory endurance, quality of life, and longevity. The extent of cardiorespiratory development (improvement in VO_{2max}) depends on the intensity, duration, and frequency of the activity. The nature of the activity often dictates the potential aerobic development. For example, jogging is much more strenuous than walking. The effort during exercise also has an impact on the degree of physiological development. The training benefits of just going through the motions of a low-impact aerobics routine, as compared to accentuating all motions (see low-impact aerobics) are of a different magnitude.

Table 4.1 includes a starting fitness level for each aerobic activity. Attempting to participate in high-intensity activities without proper conditioning often leads to discouragement and injuries. Beginners should start with low-intensity activities that have a minimum risk for injuries. In some cases, such as in high-impact aerobics and rope skipping, the risk of injuries remains high despite adequate conditioning. These activities should be used only to supplement training and are not recommended as the sole mode of exercise.

The MET range for the various activities is also included in Table 4.1. METS are an alternate method of prescribing exercise intensity and are frequently used by physicians who work with cardiac patients. One MET represents *the body's energy requirement at rest or the equivalent of an oxygen uptake of 3.5 ml/kg/min.* A 10-MET activity requires a tenfold increase in the resting energy requirement, or approximately 35 ml/kg/min. MET levels for a given activity vary according to the effort the individual expends. The harder a person exercises, the higher is the MET level.

The effectiveness of the various aerobic activities in aiding with weight management also is provided in Table 4.1. As a rule of thumb, the greater the muscle mass involved during exercise, the better are the results. Rhythmic and continuous activities that involve large amounts of muscle mass are most effective in burning calories.

Higher intensity activities increase caloric expenditure as well. Increasing exercise time, however, compensates for lower intensities. If carried out long enough (45 to 60 minutes five to six times per week), even walking can be an excellent exercise mode for weight loss. Additional information on a comprehensive weight management program is given in Chapter 6.

SKILL-RELATED FITNESS

As indicated in Chapter 1, skill-related fitness is needed for success in athletics and effective performance of lifetime sports and activities. The components of skill-related fitness are agility, balance, coordination, power, reaction time, and speed (see Chapter 1 for definitions of each component). All are important to varying degrees in sports and athletics.

For example, outstanding gymnasts must achieve good skill-related fitness in all components. A significant amount of agility is necessary to perform a double back somersault with a full twist — a skill during which the athlete must rotate simultaneously around one axis and twist around a different one. Static balance is essential for maintaining a handstand or a scale. Dynamic balance is needed to perform many of the gymnastics routines (e.g., balance beam, parallel bars, pommel horse). Coordination is important to successfully integrate various skills requiring varying degrees of difficulty into one routine. Power and speed are needed to propel

TABLE 4.1 ❖ Ratings for Aerobic Activities

Activity	Recommended Starting Fitness Level[1]	Injury Risk[2]	Potential Cardiovascular Endurance Development (VO$_{2max}$)[3,5]	Upper Body Strength Development[3]	Lower Body Strength Development[3]	Upper Body Flexibility Development[3]	Lower Body Flexibility Development[3]	Weight Control[3]	MET Level[4,5,6]	Caloric Expenditure (cal/hour)[5,6]
Walking	B	L	1–2	1	2	1	1	3	4–6	300–450
Walking, Water—Chest-Deep	I	L	2–4	2	3	1	1	3	6–10	450–750
Hiking	B	L	2–4	1	3	1	1	3	6–10	450–750
Jogging	I	M	3–5	1	3	1	1	5	6–15	450–1125
Jogging, Deep Water	A	L	3–5	2	2	1	1	5	8–15	600–1125
High-Impact Aerobics	A	H	3–4	2	4	3	2	4	6–12	450–900
Low-Impact Aerobics	B	L	2–4	2	3	3	2	3	5–10	375–750
Step Aerobics	I	M	2–4	2	3–4	3	2	3–4	5–12	375–900
Moderate-Impact Aerobics	I	M	2–4	2	3	3	2	3	6–12	450–900
Swimming (front crawl)	B	L	3–5	4	2	3	1	3	6–12	450–900
Water Aerobics	B	L	2–4	3	3	3	2	3	6–12	450–900
Stationary Cycling	B	L	2–4	1	4	1	1	3	6–10	450–750
Road Cycling	I	M	2–5	1	4	1	1	3	6–12	450–900
Cross-Training	I	M	3–5	2–3	3–4	2–3	1–2	3–5	6–15	450–1125
Rope Skipping	I	H	3–5	2	4	1	2	3–5	8–15	600–1125
Cross-Country Skiing	B	M	4–5	4	4	2	2	4–5	10–16	750–1200
Aero-belt Exercise	B	M	4–5	4	4	3	2	4–5	10–16	750–1200
In-Line Skating	I	M	2–4	2	4	2	2	3	6–10	450–750
Rowing	B	L	3–5	4	2	3	1	4	8–14	600–1050
Stair Climbing	B	L	3–5	1	4	1	1	4–5	8–15	600–1125
Racquet Sports	I	M	2–4	3	3	3	2	3	6–10	450–750

[1] B = Beginner, I = Intermediate, A = Advanced

[2] L = Low, M = Moderate, H = High

[3] 1 = Low, 2 = Fair, 3 = Average, 4 = Good, 5 = Excellent

[4] One MET represents the rate of energy expenditure at rest (3.5 ml/kg/min). Each additional MET is a multiple of the resting value. For example, 5 METs represents an energy expenditure equivalent to five times the resting value or about 17.5 ml/kg/min.

[5] Varies according to the person's effort (exercise intensity) during exercise.

[6] Varies according to body weight.

the body into the air, such as when tumbling or vaulting. Reaction time is necessary in determining when to end rotation upon a visual clue, such as spotting the floor on a dismount.

As with the health-related fitness components, the principle of specificity of training also applies to skill-related components. This principle states that to develop a given skill, the training program must be specific to the type of skill the individual is trying to achieve.

In the case of agility, balance, coordination, and reaction time, research indicates that development of these components is highly task-specific. To develop a certain task or skill, the individual must practice that same task many times. It seems to have very little crossover learning effect.

For instance, proper practice of a handstand (balance) eventually will lead to successful performance of the skill, but complete mastery of this skill does not ensure that the person will have immediate success when attempting to perform other static balance positions in gymnastics. Power and speed may be improved with a specific strength-training program or frequent repetition of the specific task to be improved, or both.

The rate of learning in skill-related fitness varies from person to person, mainly because these components seem to be determined to a large extent by hereditary factors. Individuals with good skill-related fitness tend to do better and learn faster when performing a wide variety of skills. Nevertheless, few individuals enjoy complete success in all skill-related components. Furthermore, though skill-related fitness can be enhanced with practice, improvements in reaction time and speed are limited and seem to be related primarily to genetic endowment.

Although we do not know how much skill-related fitness is desirable, everyone should attempt to develop and maintain a better than average level. While this type of fitness is crucial for athletes, it also is an important component to leading a better and happier life. Improving skill-related fitness not only affords an individual more enjoyment and success in lifetime sports (e.g., basketball, tennis, racquetball), but

it also can help a person cope more effectively in emergency situations. For example:

1. Good reaction time, balance, coordination, and agility can help you avoid a fall or break a fall and thereby minimize injury.

2. The ability to generate maximum force in a short time (power) may be crucial to ameliorate injury or even preserve life in a situation in which you may be called upon to lift a heavy object that has fallen on another person or even on yourself.

3. In our society, where the average lifespan continues to expand, maintaining speed can be especially important for elderly people. Many of them and, for that matter, many unfit/overweight young people no longer have the speed they need to cross an intersection safely before the light changes for oncoming traffic.

Regular participation in a health-related fitness program can heighten performance of skill-related components and vice versa. For example, significantly overweight people do not have good agility or speed. Because participating in aerobic and strength-training programs helps take off body fat, an overweight individual who loses weight through such an exercise program can improve agility and speed. A sound flexibility program decreases resistance to motion around body joints, which may increase agility, balance, and overall coordination. Improvements in strength definitely help develop power. On the other hand, people who have good skill-related fitness usually participate in lifetime sports and games, which in turn helps develop health-related fitness.

EVALUATING THE CONTRIBUTIONS OF SKILL-RELATED FITNESS ACTIVITIES

Similar to the fitness benefits of the aerobic activities discussed previously in this chapter and given in Table 4.1, the contributions of skill-related activities also vary among activities and individuals. The extent to which an activity helps develop each skill-related component varies not only by the effort the individual makes but, most important, by proper execution (technique) of the skill (correct coaching is highly recommended) and the individual's potential based on genetic endowment. As with aerobic activities, a summary of potential contributions to skill fitness for selected activities is provided in Table 4.2.

TEAM SPORTS

Choosing activities that you enjoy greatly enhances adherence to exercise. People tend to repeat things they enjoy doing. Enjoyment by itself is a reward. In this regard, combining individual activities (such as jogging or swimming) with team sports is fitting.

People with good skill-related fitness usually participate in lifetime sports and games, which in turn helps develop health-related fitness. Individuals who enjoyed basketball or soccer in their youth tend to stick to those activities later in life. Joining teams and community leagues may be all that is needed to stop contemplating and start participating.

The social aspect of team sports also provides added incentive to participate. Team sports offer an opportunity to interact with people who share a common interest with you. Being a member of a team creates responsibility — another incentive to exercise when you are expected to be there. Furthermore, lifetime friendships are created, strengthening the social and emotional dimensions of wellness.

For those who were not able to participate in youth sports, it's never too late to start (see the discussion of motivation and behavior modification in Chapter 1). Don't be afraid to select a new activity, even if that means learning new skills. The fitness and social rewards will be ample.

TIPS TO ENHANCE YOUR AEROBIC WORKOUT

A typical aerobic workout is divided into three parts (see Figure 4.2):

1. A 2- to 5-minute warm-up phase during which the heart rate is increased gradually to the target zone.
2. The actual aerobic workout, during which the heart rate is maintained in the target zone for 20 to 60 minutes.
3. A 5- to 10-minute aerobic cool-down, when the heart rate is lowered gradually toward the resting level.

The exerciser should not stop abruptly following aerobic exercise. It will cause blood to pool in the exercised body parts, diminishing the

TABLE 4.2 ✦ Contribution* of selected activities to skill-related components.

Activity	Agility	Balance	Coordination	Power	Reaction Time	Speed
Alpine Skiing	4	5	4	2	3	2
Archery	1	2	4	2	3	1
Badminton	4	3	4	2	4	3
Baseball	3	2	4	4	5	4
Basketball	4	3	4	3	4	3
Bowling	2	2	4	1	1	1
Cross-country Skiing	3	4	3	2	2	1
Football	4	4	4	4	4	3
Golf	1	2	5	3	1	3
Gymnastics	5	5	5	4	3	3
Ice Skating	5	5	5	3	3	3
In-line Skating	4	4	4	3	2	4
Judo/Karate	5	5	5	4	5	4
Racquetball	5	4	4	4	5	4
Soccer	5	3	5	5	3	4
Table Tennis	5	3	5	3	5	3
Tennis	4	3	5	3	5	3
Volleyball	4	3	5	4	5	3
Water Skiing	3	4	3	2	2	1
Wrestling	5	5	5	4	5	4

*1 = Low, 2 = Fair, 3 = Average, 4 = Good, 5 = Excellent

return of blood to the heart. A lower blood return can cause dizziness or faintness, or even induce cardiac abnormalities.

To monitor the target training zone, you will need to check your exercise heart rate. As described in Chapter 2, the pulse can be checked on the radial or the carotid artery. When taking the pulse at the carotid artery, too much pressure on the artery may slow the heart and produce an inaccurate measurement.

When you check the heart rate, begin with zero and count the number of beats in a 10-second period, then multiply by 6 to get the per-minute pulse rate. You should take your exercise heart rate for 10 seconds rather than a full minute because the heart rate begins to slow down 15 seconds after you stop exercising.

Feeling the pulse while exercising is difficult. Participants should stop during exercise to check the pulse. If the heart rate is too low, increase the intensity of the exercise. If the rate is too high, slow down. You may want to practice taking your pulse several times during the day to become familiar with the monitoring techniques.

For the first few weeks of your program, heart rate should be monitored several times during the exercise session. As you become familiar with your body's response to exercise, you may have to monitor the heart rate only twice — once at 5 to 7 minutes into the exercise session and a second time near the end of the workout.

Another technique sometimes used to determine your exercise intensity is simply to talk during exercise and then take the pulse immediately after that. Learning to associate the amount of difficulty when talking with the actual exercise heart rate will allow you to develop a sense of how hard you are working. Generally, if you can talk easily, you are not working hard enough. If you can talk but are slightly breathless, you should be close to the target range. If

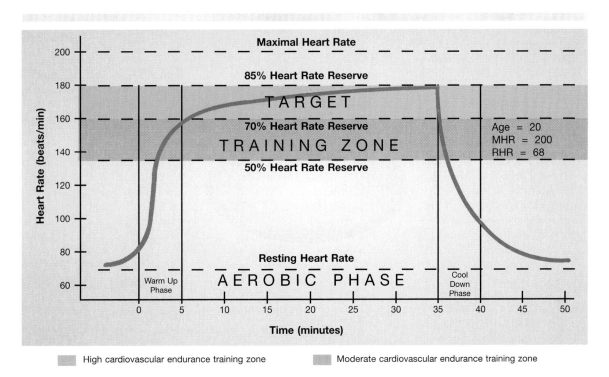

FIGURE 4.2 ❖ Typical aerobic workout pattern.

you cannot talk at all, you are working too hard.

If you have difficulty keeping up with your exercise program, you may need to reconsider your objectives and start much more slowly. Behavior modification is a process. From a physiological and psychological point of view, you may not be able to carry out an exercise session for a full 20 to 30 minutes. For the first 2 to 3 weeks, therefore, you may just want to take a few 5-minute daily walks. As your body adapts physically and mentally, you then may increase the length and intensity of the exercise sessions gradually.

As a final point, learn to listen to your body. At times you will feel unusually fatigued or have much discomfort. Pain is the body's way of letting you know something is wrong.

If you have pain or undue discomfort during or after exercise, you need to slow down or discontinue your exercise program and notify the course instructor. The instructor may be able to pinpoint the reason for the discomfort or recommend that you consult your physician. You also are going to be able to prevent potential injuries by paying attention to pain signals and making adjustments accordingly.

NOTES

1. W. D. McArdle, F. I. Katch, and V. L. Katch, *Essentials of Exercise Physiology* (Philadelphia: Lea & Febiger, 1994).

2. J. L. Christi, L. M. Sheldahl, F. E. Tristani, L. S. Wann, K. B. Sagar, S. G. Levandoski, M. J. Ptacin, K. A. Sobocinski, and R. D. Morris, "Cardiovascular Regulation During Head-out Water Immersion Exercise," *Journal of Applied Physiology*, 69 (1990), 657-664.

3. L. M. Sheldahl, F. E. Tristani, P. S. Clifford, C.V. Hughes, K. A. Sobocinski, and R. D. Morris, "Effect of Head-out Water Immersion on Cardiorespiratory Response to Dynamic Exercise," *Journal of American College of Cardiology*, 10 (1987), 1254–1258.

4. J. Svedenhang and J. Seger, "Running on Land and in Water: Comparative Exercise Physiology," *Medicine and Science in Sports and Exercise*, 24 (1992), 1155–1160.

5. W. W. K. Hoeger, "Is Water Aerobics Aerobic?" *Fitness Management*, 11 (April 1995), 29–30, 43.

6. W. Hoeger, D. Hopkins, and D. Barber, "Physiologic Responses to Maximal Treadmill Running and Water Aerobic Exercise," *National Aquatics Journal*, 11 (1995), 4–7.

7. W. W. K. Hoeger, T. S. Gibson, J. Moore, and D. R. Hopkins, "A Comparison of Selected Training Responses to Low Impact Aerobics and Water Aerobics," *National Aquatics Journal*, 9 (1993), 13–16.

8. W. W. K. Hoeger, M. L. Chupurdia, W. J. Nurge, and D. E. Van Zee, "Physiologic Responses to Step Aerobics and Aero-belt Step Aerobics," *Medicine and Science in Sports and Exercise*, 26 (1994), S43:246.

9. D. R. Hopkins, W. W. K. Hoeger, D. E. Van Zee, and W. J. Nurge, "Physiologic Responses to Aero-belt Walking." *Medicine and Science in Sports and Exercise*, 26 (1994), S43, 245.

10. W. J. Nurge, D. E. Van Zee, and W. W. K. Hoeger, "Physiologic Responses to Aero-belt Walking and Jogging," *Medicine and Science in Sports and Exercise*, 26 (1994), S43, 247.

11. E. J. Marcinick, J. Potts, G. Schlabach, S. Will, P. Dawson, and B. F. Hurley, "Effects of Strength Training on Lactate Threshold and Endurance Performance," *Medicine and Science in Sports and Exercise*, 23 (1991), 739–743.

Nutrition for Wellness

KEY TERMS

Amino acids

Anorexia nervosa

Antioxidants

Bulimia

Carbohydrates

Daily Values (DVs)

Dietary fiber

Fats

Minerals

Nutrition

Phytochemicals

Proteins

Recommended Dietary Allowances (RDA)

Vitamins

OBJECTIVES

✤ Define nutrition and describe its relationship to health and well-being.

✤ Learn the functions of nutrients in the human body.

✤ Become familiar with the various food groups and learn how to achieve a balanced diet.

✤ Understand the role of antioxidants in preventing disease.

✤ Become familiar with eating disorders, their associated medical problems, and behavior patterns.

✤ Identify myths and fallacies regarding nutrition.

*T*he science of nutrition studies the relationship of foods to optimal health and performance. Although all the answers are not in yet, scientific evidence has long linked good nutrition to overall health and well-being. Proper nutrition means that a person's diet is supplying all the essential nutrients to carry out normal tissue growth, repair, and maintenance. It also implies that the diet will provide enough substrates to produce the energy necessary for work, physical activity, and relaxation.

The typical American diet is too high in calories, sugar, fat, saturated fat, and sodium and not high enough in fiber. These factors all undermine good health. Overconsumption now is a major concern for many Americans.

Studies indicate that diet and nutrition often play a crucial role in the development and progression of chronic diseases. A diet high in saturated fat and cholesterol increases the risk for atherosclerosis and coronary heart disease. In sodium-sensitive individuals, high salt intake has been linked to high blood pressure. Some researchers believe that 30% to 50% of all cancers are diet-related. Obesity, diabetes mellitus, and osteoporosis also have been associated with faulty nutrition.

ESSENTIAL NUTRIENTS

The essential nutrients the human body requires are carbohydrates, fats, protein, vitamins, minerals, and water. Carbohydrates, fats, proteins, and water are termed macronutrients because *proportionately large amounts are needed daily.* Nutritionists refer to vitamins and minerals as micronutrients because *the body requires them in only small amounts.*

Depending on the amount of nutrients and calories, foods can be classified into high-nutrient density and low-nutrient density. *High-nutrient density* foods contain a low or moderate amount of calories but are packed with nutrients. Foods that are high in calories but contain few nutrients are of *low-nutrient density* and are commonly called "junk food."

Carbohydrates

Carbohydrates are the *major source of calories the body uses to provide energy for work, cell maintenance, and heat.* They also help regulate fat and metabolize protein. Each gram of carbohydrates provides the human body with 4 calories. The major sources of carbohydrates are breads, cereals, fruits, vegetables, and milk and other dairy products.

Carbohydrates are divided into simple carbohydrates and complex carbohydrates. *Simple carbohydrates* (such as candy, soda, and cakes) frequently are denoted as sugars and have little nutritive value. These carbohydrates are divided into monosaccharides (glucose, fructose, and galactose) and disaccharides (sucrose, lactose, and maltose). Simple carbohydrates often take the place of more nutritive foods in the diet.

Complex carbohydrates are formed when simple carbohydrate molecules link together. Two examples of complex carbohydrates are starches and dextrins. Starches are found commonly in seeds, corn, nuts, grains, roots, potatoes, and legumes. Dextrins are formed from the breakdown of large starch molecules exposed to dry heat, such as when bread is baked or cold cereals are produced. Complex carbohydrates provide many valuable nutrients and also can be an excellent source of fiber or roughage.

Dietary fiber is *a type of complex carbohydrate made up of plant material the human body cannot digest.* It is present mainly in leaves, skins, roots, and seeds. Processing and refining foods removes almost all of the natural fiber. In our daily diet the main sources of dietary fiber are whole-grain cereals and breads, fruits, and vegetables.

Fiber is important in the diet because it may help decrease the risk for cardiovascular disease and cancer. Several additional health disorders have been tied to low fiber intake, including constipation, diverticulitis, hemorrhoids, gallbladder disease, and obesity.

Fats

Fats, or lipids, are used in the body as a source of energy. They are the *most concentrated energy source.* Each gram of fat supplies 9 calories to the body. Fats also are part of the cell structure, used as stored energy and as an insulator to preserve body heat. They absorb shock, supply essential fatty acids, and carry the fat-soluble vitamins A, D, E, and K. The basic sources of fat are milk and other dairy products, and meats and alternates. Fats are classified into simple, compound, and derived fats.

Simple fats consists of a glyceride molecule linked to one, two, or three units of fatty acids.

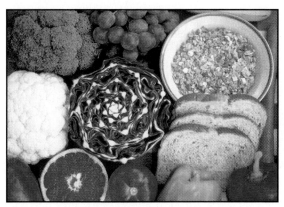
High-fiber foods are essential in a healthy diet.

According to the number of fatty acids attached, simple fats are divided into *monoglycerides* (one fatty acid), *diglycerides* (two fatty acids), and *triglycerides* (three fatty acids). More than 90% of the weight of fat in foods and more than 95% of the stored fat in the human body are in the form of triglycerides.

The length of the carbon atom chain and the amount of hydrogen saturation in fatty acids vary. Based on the extent of saturation, fatty acids are said to be saturated or unsaturated. Unsaturated fatty acids are classified further into monounsaturated and polyunsaturated fats. Saturated fatty acids are mainly of animal origin. Unsaturated fats are found mostly in plant products.

In saturated fatty acids the carbon atoms are fully saturated with hydrogens; only single bonds link the carbon atoms on the chain. These saturated fatty acids often are called saturated fats. Examples of foods high in saturated fatty acids are meats, meat fat, lard, whole milk, cream, butter, cheese, ice cream, hydrogenated oils (a process that makes oils saturated), coconut oil, and palm oils.

In *unsaturated fatty acids* (unsaturated fats), double bonds form between the unsaturated carbons. In *monounsaturated fatty acids* (MUFA) only one double bond is found along the chain. Olive, canola, rapeseed, peanut, and sesame oils are examples of monounsaturated fatty acids.

Polyunsaturated fatty acids (PUFA) contain two or more double bonds between unsaturated carbon atoms along the chain. Corn, cottonseed, safflower, walnut, sunflower, and soybean oils are high in polyunsaturated fatty acids.

Saturated fats tend to be solids that typically do not melt at room temperature. Unsaturated fats usually are liquid at room temperature. Coconut and palm oils are exceptions, as they are liquids that are high in saturated fats. Shorter fatty acid chains also tend to be liquid at room temperature.

In general, saturated fats raise the blood cholesterol level, whereas polyunsaturated and monounsaturated fats tend to lower blood cholesterol (the role of cholesterol in health and disease is discussed in Chapter 7). Polyunsaturated fats, nonetheless, also seem to cause reduction of the "good" (HDL) cholesterol, which may not really improve the cholesterol profile. Monounsaturated fats, on the other hand, seem to lower only the "bad" (LDL) cholesterol and not the good (HDL) cholesterol.

Compound fats are a combination of simple fats and other chemicals. Examples are phospholipids, glucolipids, and lipoproteins.

Derived fats combine simple and compound fats. Sterols are an example. Although sterols contain no fatty acids, they are considered lipids because they do not dissolve in water. The most often mentioned sterol is cholesterol, which is found in many foods or can be manufactured from saturated fats in the body.

Proteins

Proteins are *the main substances the body uses to build and repair tissues such as muscles, blood, internal organs, skin, hair, nails, and bones.* They are a part of hormones, enzymes, and antibodies and help maintain normal body fluid balance. Proteins also can be used as a source of energy but only if not enough carbohydrates are available. The primary sources are meats and alternates and milk and other dairy products.

The human body uses 20 amino acids, *the basic building blocks that form different types* of *protein*. Amino acids contain nitrogen, carbon, hydrogen, and oxygen. Nine of the 20 amino acids are called *essential amino acids* because the body cannot produce them. The other 11, termed *nonessential amino acids*, can be manufactured in the body if food proteins in the diet provide enough nitrogen. For normal body function all amino acids must be present at the same time.

Protein deficiency is not a problem in the usual American diet. Two glasses of skim milk combined with about 4 ounces of poultry or fish meet the daily protein requirement. Protein deficiency, however, could be a concern in some vegetarian diets. Vegetarians rely primarily on foods from the bread and cereal and fruit and vegetable groups and avoid most foods from animal sources found in the milk and meat groups. Vegetarian diets can be balanced, but this is a complicated issue that cannot be covered in a few paragraphs. Those who are interested in vegetarian diets should consult other resources.

Vitamins

Vitamins are *organic substances essential for normal bodily metabolism, growth, and development*. Vitamins function as antioxidants, as coenzymes (primarily the B complex), which regulate the work of the enzymes; and vitamin D even functions as a hormone.

Based on their solubility, vitamins are classified into two types: *fat-soluble vitamins* (A, D, E, and K) and *water-soluble vitamins* (B complex and C). The body cannot manufacture vitamins. They can be obtained only through a well-balanced diet. Additional information on the importance of antioxidant vitamins is presented later in this chapter.

Minerals

Minerals are *inorganic elements, found in the body and in food*, that serve several important functions. Minerals are constituents of all cells, especially those in hard parts of the body (bones, nails, teeth). They are crucial in maintaining water balance and the acid-base balance. They are essential components of respiratory pigments, enzymes, and enzyme systems, and they regulate muscular and nervous tissue excitability.

Water

Water is the most important nutrient, *involved in almost every vital body process*. Water is used in digesting and absorbing food, in the circulatory process, in removing waste products, in building and rebuilding cells, and in transporting other nutrients. Water is contained in almost all foods but primarily in liquid foods, fruits, and vegetables. Besides the natural content in foods, every person should drink eight to ten glasses of fluids a day.

A BALANCED DIET

Most people would like to live life to its fullest, have good health, and lead a productive life. One of the fundamental ways to do this is through a well-balanced diet. As illustrated in Figure 5.1, the recommended guidelines state that daily caloric intake should be distributed so about 58% of the total calories come from carbohydrates (48% complex carbohydrates and 10% sugar), less than 30% of the total calories from fat (equally divided [10% each] among saturated, monounsaturated, and polyunsaturated fats), and 12% of the total calories from protein (0.8 grams of protein per kilogram [2.2 pounds] of body weight). The diet also must include all the essential vitamins, minerals, and water.

One of the most detrimental health habits facing the American people today is the large amount of fat in the diet. Fat consumption in the average diet is about 37% of the total caloric intake; 30% or lower is recommended. To decrease the risk for disease, particularly cardiovascular disease and cancer, people must make a deliberate effort to decrease total fat intake. Being able to identify sources of fat in the diet is imperative to decrease fat intake.

Current

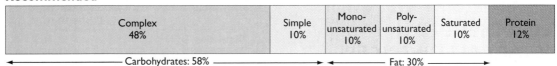

Complex 24%	Simple 27%	Mono-unsaturated 12%	Poly-unsaturated 12%	Saturated 13%	Protein 12%

◄──────── Carbohydrates: 51% ────────► ◄──────── Fat: 37% ────────►

Recommended

Complex 48%	Simple 10%	Mono-unsaturated 10%	Poly-unsaturated 10%	Saturated 10%	Protein 12%

◄──────── Carbohydrates: 58% ────────► ◄──────── Fat: 30% ────────►

FIGURE 5.1 ✤ Current and recommended distribution of fat, carbohydrate, and protein intake.

As illustrated in Figure 5.2, each gram of carbohydrates and protein supplies the body with 4 calories, and fat provides 9 calories per gram consumed (alcohol yields 7 calories per gram). In this regard, just looking at the total amount of grams consumed for each type of food can be misleading.

For example, a person who consumes 160 grams of carbohydrates, 100 grams of fat, and 70 grams of protein has a total intake of 330 grams of food. This indicates that 33% of the total grams of food is in the form of fat (100 grams of fat ÷ 330 grams of total food × 100).

In reality, almost half of the diet consists of fat calories. In this sample diet 640 calories are derived from carbohydrates (160 grams × 4 calories/gram), 280 calories from protein (70 grams × 4 calories/gram), and 900 calories from fat (100 grams × 9 calories/gram), for a total of 1,820 calories. If 900 calories are derived from fat, you can see that almost half of the total caloric intake is in the form of fat (900 ÷ 1,820 × 100 = 49.5%).

Realizing that each gram of fat equals 9 calories is a useful guideline when figuring out the fat content of individual foods. As shown in Figure 5.3, all you need to do is multiply the

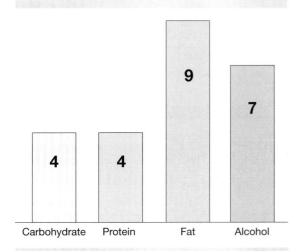

FIGURE 5.2 ✤ Caloric value (calories) per gram of food.

Servings = 120 calories	Fat = 5 g

Percent Fat Calories = (g of fat × 9) ÷ calories per serving × 100

5 g of fat × 9 calories per g of fat = 45 calories from fat

45 calories from fat ÷ 120 calories per serving × 100 = 38% fat

FIGURE 5.3 ✤ Determining percent fat calories from food.

grams of fat by 9 and divide by the total calories in that specific food. Multiply that number by 100 to get the percentage. For example, if a food label lists a total of 100 calories and 7 grams of fat, the fat content is 63% of total calories. This simple guideline can help you decrease fat in your diet.

RECOMMENDED DIETARY ALLOWANCES AND DAILY VALUES

Every 10 years or so the National Academy of Sciences issues new Recommended Dietary Allowances (RDA) based on a review of the most current research on nutrient needs of healthy people. The RDA provides *daily nutrient intake recommendations*, usually set high enough to encompass 97.5% of the healthy population in the United States. Stated another way, the RDA recommendation for any nutrient is well above almost everyone's actual requirement.

Between the late 1960s and the early 1990s, nutrient information on labels was expressed in terms of the U.S. Recommended Daily Allowances (U.S. RDA) — a set of standard values for the average consumer — derived from the 1968 edition of the RDA. In 1993 the Food and Drug Administration (FDA) revised food labeling regulations and replaced the U.S. RDA with Daily Values (DV). The main difference between the U.S. RDA and the DV is that the latter *provide the percentage of recommended daily amounts* of not just vitamins and minerals but also total fat, saturated fat, cholesterol, sodium, carbohydrates, fiber, and sugar. These daily values are based on a 2,000-calorie diet and may require adjustments depending on an individual's daily caloric needs.

The DV label (Figure 5.4) is a better guide for planning a daily diet. For example, if the DV for carbohydrates in a given meal adds up to only 35%, you know that several additional high-carbohydrate food items are required throughout that day to reach the 100% DV.

Nutrition Facts

Serving Size 1 cup (240 ml)
Servings Per Container 4

Amount Per Serving

Calories 120	Calories from Fat 45

	% Daily Value*
Total Fat 5g	8%
Saturated Fat 3g	15%
Cholesterol 20mg	7%
Sodium 120mg	5%
Total Carbohydrate 12g	4%
Dietary Fiber 0g	0%
Sugars 12g	
Protein 8g	

Vitamin A	10%	•	Vitamin C	4%
Calcium	30%	•	Iron	0%

* Percent Daily Values are based on a 2,000 calorie diet. Your daily values may be higher or lower depending on your calorie needs:

	Calories	2,000	2,500
Total Fat	Less than	65g	80g
Sat Fat	Less than	20g	25g
Cholesterol	Less than	300mg	300mg
Sodium	Less than	2,400mg	2,400mg
Total Carbohydrate		300g	375g
Fiber		25g	30g

Calories per gram:
Fat 9 • Carbohydrate 4 • Protein 4

FIGURE 5.4 ❖ Current food label using daily values (DVs).

Further, if the DV for fat from another food item is 60% or 70%, you should limit your fat intake during the rest of that day.

Both the RDA and the DV apply only to healthy people. They are not intended for people who are ill and may require additional nutrients or dietary adjustments.

NUTRIENT ANALYSIS

Achieving and maintaining a balanced diet is not as difficult as most people think. The Food Guide Pyramid contained in Figure 5.5, published by the U.S. Department of Agriculture, provides simple and sound instructions for nutrition. The pyramid contains five major food groups, along with fats, oils, and sweets, which are to be used sparingly. The daily recommended number of servings of the five major food groups are:

1. Six to 11 servings of the bread, cereal, rice, and pasta group.
2. Three to five servings of the vegetable group.
3. Two to four servings of the fruit group.
4. Two to three servings of the milk, yogurt, and cheese group.
5. Two to three servings of the meat, poultry, fish, dry beans, eggs, and nuts group.

As illustrated in the Food Guide Pyramid (Figure 5.5), grains, vegetables, and fruits provide the nutritional foundation for a healthy diet. Fruits and vegetables should include as a daily minimum one good source of vitamin A (apricots, cantaloupe, broccoli, carrots, pumpkin, dark leafy vegetables) and one good source of vitamin C (citrus fruit, kiwi fruit, cantaloupe, strawberries, broccoli, cabbage, cauliflower, green pepper).

An entirely new field of research with *promising results in disease prevention*, especially in the fight against cancer, is in the area of phytochemicals[1] ("phyto" comes from the Greek word for plant). These compounds, just recently discovered by scientists, are found in large quantities in fruits and vegetables.

The main function of phytochemicals in plants is to protect them from sunlight. In humans, however, they seem to have a powerful ability to block the formation of cancerous tumors. Their actions are so diverse that, at almost every stage of cancer, phytochemicals have the ability to block, disrupt, slow down, or even reverse the process (also see Chapter 7). These compounds are not found in pills. The message here is to eat a diet with ample fruits and vegetables. The recommendation of five to nine servings of fruits and vegetables daily has absolutely no substitute. People can't expect to eat a poor diet, pop a few pills, and derive the same benefits.

Milk, poultry, fish, and meats are to be consumed in moderation. Skim milk and low-fat milk products are recommended. Three ounces daily of poultry, fish, or meat are advised, and no more than 6 ounces per day. All visible fat and skin should be trimmed off meats and poultry before cooking. A person should eat no more than three eggs per week.

The difficult part for most people is retraining themselves to adopt a lifetime healthy nutrition plan. If you (a) avoid excessive fats, oils, sweets, alcohol, and sodium, (b) increase your fiber intake, and (c) eat the minimum number of servings recommended for each of the five major groups in the Food Pyramid, you can achieve a well-balanced diet.

To aid you in balancing your diet, a form is given in Figure 5.6 for you to record your daily food intake. First, make as many copies as the number of days you wish to analyze. Whenever you eat something, record the food and amount eaten. Recording this information immediately after each meal will enable you to keep track of your actual food intake more easily.

At the end of each day, consult the list of foods in Appendix E and record the code and number of calories for all foods consumed. Referring to Figure 5.6, record the number of servings under the respective food groups. If you eat twice the amount of a standard serving, double the calories and the number of servings.

You can evaluate your diet by checking whether you ate the minimum required servings for each food group. If you meet the minimum required servings at the end of each day, you are doing quite well in balancing your diet.

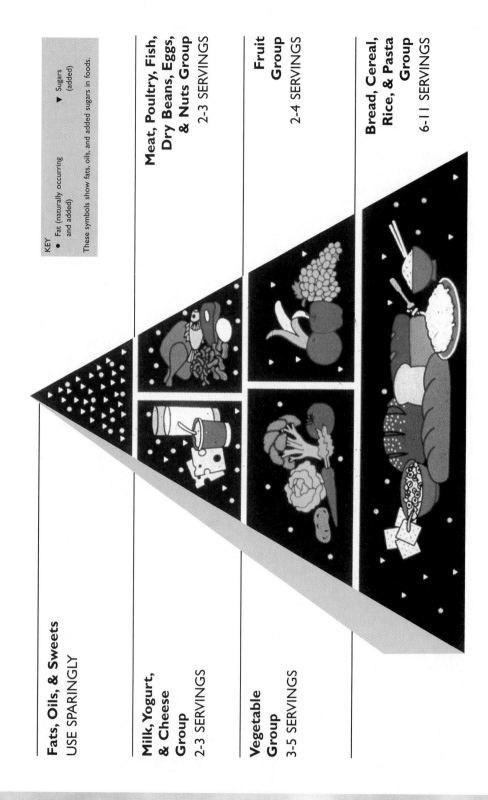

Fats, Oils, & Sweets
USE SPARINGLY

KEY
● Fat (naturally occurring and added)
▼ Sugars (added)

These symbols show fats, oils, and added sugars in foods.

Milk, Yogurt, & Cheese Group
2-3 SERVINGS

Meat, Poultry, Fish, Dry Beans, Eggs, & Nuts Group
2-3 SERVINGS

Vegetable Group
3-5 SERVINGS

Fruit Group
2-4 SERVINGS

Bread, Cereal, Rice, & Pasta Group
6-11 SERVINGS

What counts as one serving?

Breads, Cereals, Rice, and Pasta
1 slice of bread
1/2 cup of cooked rice or pasta
1/2 cup of cooked cereal
1 ounce of ready-to-eat cereal

Vegetables
1/2 cup of chopped raw or cooked vegetables
1 cup of leafy raw vegetables

Fruits
1 piece of fruit or melon wedge
3/4 cup of juice
1/2 cup of canned fruit
1/4 cup of dried fruit

Milk, Yogurt, and Cheese
1 cup of milk or yogurt
1½ to 2 ounces of cheese

Meat, Poultry, Fish, Dry Beans, Eggs, and Nuts
2½ to 3 ounces of cooked lean meat, poultry, or fish
Count 1/2 cup of cooked beans, or 1 egg, or 2 tablespoons of peanut butter as 1 ounce of lean meat (about 1/3 serving)

Fats, Oils, and Sweets
LIMIT CALORIES FROM THESE especially if you need to lose weight

The amount you eat may be more than one serving. For example, a dinner portion of spaghetti would count as two or three servings of pasta.

A Closer Look at Fat and Added Sugars

The small tip of the Pyramid shows fats, oils, and sweets. These are foods such as salad dressings, cream, butter, margarine, sugars, soft drinks, candies, and sweet desserts. Alcoholic beverages are also part of this group. These foods provide calories but few vitamins and minerals. Most people should go easy on foods from this group.

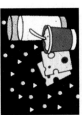
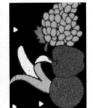

Some fat or sugar symbols are shown in the other food groups. That's to remind you that some foods in these groups can also be high in fat and added sugars, such as cheese or ice cream from the milk group, or french fries from the vegetable group. When choosing foods for a healthful diet, consider the fat and added sugars in your choices from all the food groups, not just fats, oils, and sweets from the Pyramid tip.

How many servings do you need each day?

	Women & some older adults	Children, teen girls, active women, most men	Teen boys & active men
Calorie level*	about 1,600	about 2,200	about 2,800
Bread group	6	9	11
Vegetable group	3	4	5
Fruit group	2	3	4
Milk group	2–3**	2–3**	**2–3
Meat group	2, for a total of 5 ounces	2, for a total of 6 ounces	3, for a total of 7 ounces

* These are the calorie levels if you choose lowfat, lean foods from the 5 major food groups and use foods from the fats, oils, and sweets group sparingly.

** Women who are pregnant or breastfeeding, teenagers, and young adults to age 24 need 3 servings.

*Developed by the U.S. Department of Agriculture to promote a healthy diet for people in the United States.

FIGURE 5.5 ✤ The Food Guide Pyramid: A Guide to Daily Food Choices.

In addition to meeting the daily serving guidelines, a complete nutrient analysis is recommended to rate your diet accurately. A nutrient analysis can pinpoint potential problem areas in your diet, such as too much fat, saturated fat, cholesterol, sodium, and the like. A complete nutrient analysis can be quite an educational experience because most people do not realize how detrimental and non-nutritious many common foods are.

Analyzing your diet is quite simple if you utilize the computer software for this analysis.* To conduct the analysis, use the information you have recorded already on the form provided in Figure 5.6. Before running the software, fill out the information at the top of this form (age, weight, sex, activity rating, and number of days to be analyzed) and make sure the foods are recorded by the code and standard amounts given in the list of selected foods in Appendix E. Using the software, up to 7 days may be analyzed. The analysis covers calories, carbohydrates, fats, cholesterol, and sodium, as well as eight crucial nutrients: protein, calcium, iron, vitamin A, thiamin, riboflavin, niacin, and vitamin C. If the diet has enough of these eight nutrients, the foods (in natural form) consumed to provide these nutrients typically contain all the other nutrients the human body needs.

The computer-generated printout also includes the average daily nutrient intake and the recommended dietary allowance (RDA) comparison for all the above nutrients. A sample nutrient analysis printout is provided in Figure 5.7, at the end of the chapter.

NUTRIENT SUPPLEMENTATION

Four of every 10 adults in the United States take nutrient supplements daily. RDA vitamin and mineral requirements for the body, however, can be met by consuming as few as 1,200 calories per day, as long as the diet contains the recommended servings from the five food groups.

For most people, excessive vitamin and mineral supplementation is unnecessary and sometimes is unsafe. Iron deficiency (determined through blood testing) is an exception for women who have heavy menstrual flow. Some pregnant and lactating women also may require supplements. In these instances, supplements should be taken under a physician's supervision.

Other people who may benefit from supplementation are alcoholics and street-drug users who do not have a balanced diet, smokers, strict vegetarians, individuals on extremely low-calorie diets, elderly people who don't eat balanced meals regularly, and newborn infants (usually given a single dose of vitamin K to prevent abnormal bleeding).

Antioxidants: Free Radical Combatants

Much research currently is being done to study the effects of antioxidant supplements in thwarting several chronic diseases. Vitamins C, E, beta-carotene, *a precursor to vitamin A,* and the mineral selenium serve as antioxidants, preventing oxygen from combining with other substances it may damage (see Table 5.1). Oxygen is utilized during metabolism to change carbohydrates and fats into energy. During this process oxygen is transformed into stable forms of water and carbon dioxide. A small amount of oxygen, however, ends up in an unstable form, referred to as free radicals.

A free radical molecule has a normal proton nucleus with a single unpaired electron. Having only one electron makes the free radical extremely reactive, and it constantly looks to pair the electron up with one from another molecule. When a free radical steals the second electron from another molecule, that other molecule in turn becomes a free radical. This chain reaction goes on until two free radicals meet to form a stable molecule. Antioxidants help stabilize free radicals so they will not be as reactive until a match can be found.

---

* Your instructor may have a copy of this software, available through Morton Publishing Company in Englewood, Colorado.

Date: _____

Name: _____ Age: _____ Weight: _____ lbs.

Sex: _____ M _____ F   (Pregnant – P, Lactating – L, Neither – N)

Activity Rating: Sedentary (limited physical activity)   = 1
                   Moderate physical activity   = 2
                   Hard labor (strenuous physical activity)   = 3

Number of days to be analyzed: _____   Day: _____ (1, 2 . . .)

No.	Code*	Food	Amount	Calories	Bread, Cereal, Rice & Pasta	Vegetable	Fruit	Milk, Yogurt & Cheese	Meat, Poultry, Fish, Dry Beans, Eggs, & Nuts
									Food Groups
1									
2									
3									
4									
5									
6									
7									
8									
9									
10									
11									
12									
13									
14									
15									
16									
17									
18									
19									
20									
21									
22									
23									
24									
25									
26									
27									
28									
29									
30									
Totals									
Recommended Servings				**	6–11	3–5	2–4	2–3	2–3
Deficiencies									

*See list of nutritive value of selected foods in Appendix E.
**See Table 5.1.

FIGURE 5.6 ❖ Daily diet record form.

Date: _____

Name: _____ Age: _____ Weight: _____ lbs.

Sex: _____ M _____ F   (Pregnant – P, Lactating – L, Neither – N)

Activity Rating: Sedentary (limited physical activity)   = 1
                    Moderate physical activity   = 2
                    Hard labor (strenuous physical activity)   = 3

Number of days to be analyzed: _____   Day: _____ (1, 2 . . .)

No.	Code*	Food	Amount	Calories	Bread, Cereal, Rice & Pasta	Vegetable	Fruit	Milk, Yogurt & Cheese	Meat, Poultry, Fish, Dry Beans, Eggs, & Nuts
1									
2									
3									
4									
5									
6									
7									
8									
9									
10									
11									
12									
13									
14									
15									
16									
17									
18									
19									
20									
21									
22									
23									
24									
25									
26									
27									
28									
29									
30									
Totals									
Recommended Servings				**	6–11	3–5	2–4	2–3	2–3
Deficiencies									

*See list of nutritive value of selected foods in Appendix E.
**See Table 5.1

FIGURE 5.6 ♣ Daily diet record form (continued).

TABLE 5.1 ✤ Antioxidant Content of Selected Foods

Nutrient	Good Sources	Antioxidant Effect
Vitamin C	Citrus fruit, kiwi fruit, cantaloupe, strawberries, broccoli, green or red peppers, cauliflower, cabbage	Appears to inactivate oxygen free radicals
Vitamin E	Vegetable oils, yellow and green leafy vegetables, margarine, wheatgerm, oatmeal, almonds, and whole grain breads, cereals	Protects lipids from oxidation
Beta-carotene	Carrots, squash, pumpkin, sweet potatoes, broccoli, green leafy vegetables	Soaks up oxygen free radicals
Selenium	Seafood, meat, whole grains	Helps prevent damage to cell structures

Free radicals attack and damage proteins and lipids, in particular the cell membrane and DNA. This damage is thought to contribute to the development of conditions such as cardiovascular disease, cancer, emphysema, cataracts, Parkinson's disease, and premature aging (also see Chapter 7). Solar radiation, cigarette smoke, radiation, and other environmental factors also seem to encourage the formation of free radicals. Antioxidants are thought to offer protection by absorbing free radicals before they can cause damage and also by interrupting the sequence of reactions once damage has begun, thwarting certain chronic diseases.

Antioxidants are found abundantly in food, especially in fruits and vegetables. Unfortunately, only 9% of Americans eat the minimum five daily servings of fruits and vegetables[2] (5 to 9 are recommended).

In a departure from past recommendations, in 1994 the editorial board of the University of California at Berkeley *Wellness Letter* issued the following antioxidant supplementation guidelines for people who eat at least five daily servings of antioxidant-rich fruits and vegetables:[3]

✤ 250 to 500 mg of vitamin C.

✤ 200 to 800 IU of vitamin E.

✤ 10,000 to 25,000 IU of beta-carotene.

In a special report, the editorial board also issued the following statement:[4]

> The editorial board of the Wellness Letter has been reluctant to recommend supplementary vitamins on a broad scale for healthy people eating healthy diets. But the accumulation of research in recent years has caused us to change our minds.

Based on these recommendations, people who consume nine ample amounts of fresh fruits and vegetables daily could get their daily beta-carotene and vitamin C requirements through the diet. To obtain the recommended guideline for vitamin E through diet alone, however, is practically impossible. As shown in Table 5.2, vitamin E is not easily found in large quantities in foods typically consumed in the diet. Thus, supplements are encouraged. When supplements (in general) are taken, they should be taken with meals and split in two to three doses per day.[5]

Supplements of the mineral selenium are not recommended at this point, although one Brazil

TABLE 5.2 ❖ Antioxidant Content of Selected Foods

Beta-Carotene	IU
Apricot (1 medium)	675
Broccoli (½ cup, frozen)	1,740
Broccoli (½ cup, raw)	680
Cantaloupe (1 cup)	5,160
Carrot, (1 medium, raw)	20,255
Green peas (½ cup, frozen)	535
Mango (1 medium)	8,060
Mustard greens (½ cup, frozen)	3,350
Papaya (1 medium)	6,120
Spinach (½ cup, frozen)	7,395
Sweet potato (1 medium, baked)	24,875
Tomato (1 medium)	1,395
Turnip greens (½ cup, boiled)	3,960

Vitamin C	mg
Acerola (1 cup, raw)	1,640
Acerola juice (8 oz)	3,864
Cantaloupe (½ melon, medium)	90
Cranberry juice (8 oz)	90
Grapefruit (½, medium, white)	52
Grapefruit juice (8 oz)	92
Guava (1 medium)	165
Kiwi (1 medium)	75
Lemon juice (8 oz)	110
Orange (1 medium)	66
Orange juice (8 oz)	120
Papaya (1 medium)	85
Pepper (½ cup, red, chopped, raw)	95
Strawberries (1 cup, raw)	88

Vitamin E	IU	mg*
Almond oil (1 tbsp)		5.3
Almonds (1 oz)	10.1	
Canola oil (1 tbsp)		9.0
Cottonseed oil (1 tbsp)		5.2
Hazelnuts (1 oz)	4.4	
Kale (1 cup)	15.0	
Margarine (1 tbsp)		2.0
Peanuts (1 oz)	3.0	
Shrimp (3 oz, boiled)	3.1	
Sunflower seeds (1 oz, dry)	14.2	
Sunflower seed oil (1 tbsp)		6.9
Sweet potato (1 medium, baked)	7.2	
Wheat germ oil (1 tbsp)		20.0

* Vitamin E values for oils are commonly expressed in milligrams (mg). One mg is almost equal to 1 IU.

nut per day seems to provide the necessary amount of antioxidant for this nutrient. Five or more daily Brazil nuts per day can lead to toxic levels of this mineral in the body.[6]

Although not an antioxidant, folacin (a B vitamin) also is recommended (400 mcg) for all premenopausal women.[7] Folacin helps prevent certain birth defects and seems to offer protection against colon and cervical cancers.

Toxic effects with antioxidant supplementation are rare when taken in the previously recommended amounts. Generally, up to 4,000 mg of vitamin C, 3,200 IU of vitamin E, and 50,000 IU of beta-carotene seem safe. If you experience any of the following side effects, stop supplementation and check with your physician:

❖ Vitamin E: Gastrointestinal disturbances, increase in blood lipids.

❖ Vitamin C: Nausea, diarrhea, abdominal cramps, kidney stones, liver problems.

❖ Beta-carotene: Although not harmful, yellow pigmentation of the skin.

❖ Selenium: Vomiting, diarrhea, irritability, fatigue, lesions of the skin and nervous tissue, loss of hair and nails.

Large supplements of vitamin E are not recommended for individuals on anticoagulant therapy. Vitamin E is in itself an anticoagulant. Check with your physician if you are on such therapy. Pregnant women need a physician's approval prior to beta-carotene supplementation. It also may be unsafe if taken with alcohol and by people who drink more than 4 ounces of pure alcohol per day (the equivalent of 8 beers).

A few researchers are expressing concern for people who participate regularly in high-intensity exercise (above 70% of heart rate reserve — see Chapter 3) or prolonged exercise (more than 5 hours per week). Overtraining increases the production of free radicals and well may exceed the body's antioxidant defense mechanism. This high amount of free radicals may increase the risk for chronic diseases, including cancer.[8]

Scientists, therefore, are examining a possible link between "heavy" exercise and disease in people who otherwise lead a healthy lifestyle. Although the research is scarce, Dr. Kenneth Cooper, in his book *Antioxidant Revolution*, recommends higher doses of antioxidants for athletes and heavy exercisers: 3,000 mg of vitamin C, 1,200 IU of vitamin E, and 50,000 IU of beta-carotene.[9] Awareness of side effects is important if these higher amounts are taken.

Many people who regularly eat foods high in fat content or too many sweets think they need supplementation to balance their diet. This is another fallacy about nutrition. The problem in these cases is not necessarily a lack of vitamins and minerals but, instead, a diet too high in calories, fat, and sodium. Supplements are no substitute for a well-balanced diet.

Wholesome foods contain vitamins, minerals, carbohydrates, fiber, proteins, fats, phytochemicals, and others not yet discovered. Researchers do not know if the protective effects are caused by the antioxidants themselves, in combination with other nutrients (such as phytochemicals), or actually by some other nutrients in food that have not been investigated yet. Many nutrients work in synergy, enhancing chemical processes in the body. Supplementation will not offset poor eating habits. Pills are no substitute for common sense.

DISORDERED EATING

Anorexia nervosa and bulimia are physical and emotional problems thought to develop from individual, family, or social pressures. These disorders are characterized by an intense fear of becoming fat, which does not disappear even when losing extreme amounts of weight. Anorexia nervosa and bulimia are increasing steadily in most industrialized nations where society encourages low-calorie diets and thinness.

Anorexia Nervosa

Anorexia nervosa is *a condition of self-imposed starvation to lose and then maintain very low body weight*. Approximately 19 of every 20

anorexics are young women. An estimated 1% of the female population in the United States is anorexic. Anorexic individuals seem to fear weight gain more than death from starvation. Furthermore, they have a distorted image of their body and think of themselves as being fat even when they are emaciated.

Although a genetic predisposition may contribute, the anorexic person often comes from a mother-dominated home, with possible drug addictions in the family. The syndrome may emerge following a stressful life event and uncertainty about one's ability to cope efficiently.

Because the female role in society is changing more rapidly, women seem to be especially susceptible. Life experiences such as gaining weight, starting the menstrual period, beginning college, losing a boyfriend, having poor self-esteem, being socially rejected, starting a professional career, or becoming a wife or a mother may trigger the syndrome.

These individuals typically begin a diet and at first feel in control and happy about the weight loss, even if they are not overweight. To speed up the weight loss, they frequently combine extreme dieting with exhaustive exercise and overuse of laxatives and diuretics.

Anorexics commonly develop obsessive and compulsive behaviors and emphatically deny their condition. They are preoccupied with food, meal planning, grocery shopping, and unusual eating habits. As they lose weight and their health begins to deteriorate, anorexics feel weak and tired and may realize they have a problem but will not stop the starvation and refuse to consider the behavior as abnormal.

Once they have lost a lot of weight and malnutrition sets in, physical changes become more visible. Some typical changes are amenorrhea (stopping menstruation), digestive problems, extreme sensitivity to cold, hair and skin problems, fluid and electrolyte abnormalities (which may lead to an irregular heartbeat and sudden stopping of the heart), injuries to nerves and tendons, abnormalities of immune function, anemia, growth of fine body hair, mental confusion, inability to concentrate, lethargy, depression, skin dryness, lower skin and body temperature, and osteoporosis.

Diagnostic criteria for anorexia nervosa are:[10]

❖ Refusal to maintain body weight over a minimal normal weight for age and height (e.g., weight loss leading to maintenance of body weight 15% below that expected; or failure to make expected weight gain during period of growth, leading to body weight 15% below that expected).

❖ Intense fear of gaining weight or becoming fat, even though underweight.

❖ Disturbance in the way in which one's body weight, size, or shape is experienced (e.g., the person claims to "feel fat" even when emaciated or believes that one area of the body is "too fat" even when obviously underweight).

❖ In females, absence of at least three consecutive menstrual cycles when otherwise expected to occur (primary or secondary amen-orrhea). (A woman is considered to have amenorrhea if her periods occur only following hormone therapy, e.g., estrogen administration.)

Many of the changes induced by anorexia nervosa can be reversed. Treatment almost always requires professional help, and the sooner it is started, the better are the chances for reversibility and cure. Therapy consists of a combination of medical and psychological techniques to restore proper nutrition, prevent medical complications, and modify the environment or events that triggered the syndrome.

Seldom are anorexics able to overcome the problem by themselves. Unfortunately, they strongly deny their condition. They are able to hide it and deceive friends and relatives quite effectively. Based on their behavior, many of them meet all of the characteristics of anorexia nervosa, but it goes undetected because both thinness and dieting are socially acceptable. Only a well-trained clinician is able to make a positive diagnosis.

Bulimia

A pattern of binge eating and purging, bulimia is more prevalent than anorexia nervosa. For many years it was thought to be a variant of anorexia nervosa, but now it is identified as a separate condition. It afflicts mainly young people. As many as one in every five women on college campuses may be bulimic, according to some estimates. Bulimia also is more prevalent than anorexia nervosa in males.

Bulimics usually are healthy-looking people, well-educated, near recommended body weight, and seem to enjoy food and often socialize around it. In actuality, they are emotionally insecure, rely on others, and lack self-confidence and self-esteem. Recommended weight and food are important to them.

The binge-purge cycle usually occurs in stages. As a result of stressful life events or the simple compulsion to eat, bulimics engage periodically in binge eating that may last an hour or longer.

With some apprehension, bulimics anticipate and plan the cycle. Next they feel an urgency to begin, followed by large and uncontrollable food consumption during which they may eat several thousand calories (up to 10,000 calories in extreme cases). After a short period of relief and satisfaction, feelings of deep guilt, shame, and intense fear of gaining weight ensue. Purging seems to be an easy answer, as the binging cycle can continue without fear of gaining weight.

The diagnostic criteria for bulimia are:[11]

❖ Recurrent episodes of binge eating (rapid consumption of a large amount of food in a discrete period of time).

❖ A feeling of lack of control over eating behavior during the eating binges.

❖ Regular practice of self-induced vomiting or use of laxatives or diuretics, or strict dieting or fasting, or vigorous exercise to prevent weight gain.

❖ A minimum average of two binge eating episodes a week for at least 3 months.

- Persistent overconcern with body shape and weight.

The most typical form of purging is self-induced vomiting. Bulimics, too, frequently ingest strong laxatives and emetics. Near-fasting diets and strenuous bouts of exercise are common. Medical problems associated with bulimia include cardiac arrhythmias, amenorrhea, kidney and bladder damage, ulcers, colitis, tearing of the esophagus or stomach, tooth erosion, gum damage, and general muscular weakness.

Unlike anorexics, bulimics realize their behavior is abnormal and feel great shame about it. Fearing social rejection, they pursue the binge-purge cycle in secrecy and at unusual hours of the day.

Bulimia can be treated successfully when the person realizes that this destructive behavior is not the solution to life's problems. A change in attitude can prevent permanent damage or death.

Treatment for anorexia nervosa and bulimia are available on most school campuses through the school's counseling center or the health center. Local hospitals also offer treatment for these conditions. Many communities have support groups, frequently led by professional personnel and usually free of charge.

SOUND NUTRITION: A LIFETIME COMMITMENT FOR WELLNESS ENHANCEMENT

Proper nutrition, a sound exercise program, and quitting smoking (for those who smoke) are the three factors that do the most for health, longevity, and quality of life. Achieving and maintaining a balanced diet is not as difficult as most people would think. The difficult part for most people is retraining themselves to follow a lifetime healthy nutrition plan — a diet that includes lots of grains, legumes, fruits, vegetables, and low-fat dairy products, with moderate use of animal protein, junk food, sodium, and alcohol.

In spite of the ample scientific evidence linking poor dietary habits to early disease and mortality rates, most people are not willing to change their eating patterns. Even when faced with obesity, elevated blood lipids, hypertension, and other nutrition-related conditions, most people do not change. The motivating factor to change one's eating habits seems to be a major health breakdown, such as a heart attack, a stroke, or cancer.

An ounce of prevention is worth a pound of cure. The sooner you implement the dietary guidelines presented in this chapter, the better will be your chances of preventing chronic diseases and reaching a higher state of wellness.

NOTES

1. S. Begley. "Beyond Vitamins," *Newsweek*, April 25, 1994, pp. 45–49.
2. "Vitamin Report," University of California at Berkeley *Wellness Letter* (Palm Coast, FL: The editors, October, 1994).
3. "Antioxidants: Never Too Late," University of California at Berkeley *Wellness Letter*, 10:8 (1994), 2.
4. "Vitamin Report."
5. S. Kalish, "The Free Radical Radical: Kenneth Cooper, M.D., on Antioxidants and the Dangers of Hard Running." *Running Times*, March 1995, 16-17.
6. J. Carper. "Say 'Nuts' to Heart Disease," *USA Weekend*, December 2–4, 1994, 8–9.
7. "Vitamin Report."
8. K. H. Cooper, *Antioxidant Revolution* (Nashville, TN: Thomas Nelson Publishers, 1994).
9. Cooper.
10. American Psychiatric Association, *Diagnostic and Statistical Manual of Mental Disorders*. (Washington, DC: APA, 1987), p. 67.
11. APA.

Jane R. Moore   Date: 02-12-1992
Age: 20
Body Weight: 141 lbs (64.0 kg)
Activity Rating: Moderate

Food Intake Day One

Food	Amount	Calo-ries	Pro-tein gm	Fat gm	Sat Fat gm	Cho-les-terol mg	Car-bohy-drate gm	Cal-cium mg	Iron mg	Sodium mg	Vit A I.U.	Thi-amin mg	Ribo-fla-vin mg	Nia-cin mg	Vit C mg
Cocoa/hot/with whole milk	1 cup	218	9.1	9	6.1	33	26	298	0.8	123	318	0.10	0.44	0.4	2
Egg/scrambled w/milk butter	1 egg(s)	95	6.0	7	3.0	282	1	54	0.9	176	510	0.04	0.18	0.0	0
Bread/white	2 slice(s)	136	4.4	2	0.4	0	26	42	1.2	254	0	0.12	0.10	1.2	0
Butter	2 tsp	72	0.0	8	0.8	24	0	2	0.0	92	320	0.00	0.00	0.0	0
Milk/whole	1 c	159	9.0	9	5.1	34	12	288	0.1	120	350	0.07	0.40	0.2	2
Bread/whole wheat	2 slice(s)	122	5.2	2	1.2	0	24	50	1.6	264	0	0.12	0.06	1.4	0
Tuna/canned/oil/drained	1.5 oz.	84	12.5	4	0.9	30	0	4	0.8	69	35	0.02	0.05	5.1	0
Mayonnaise	2 tsp.	72	0.0	8	1.4	6	0	2	0.0	56	26	0.00	0.00	0.0	0
Pickles/dill	1 large	15	0.9	0	0.0	0	3	35	1.4	1,928	140	0.00	0.03	0.0	8
Potato/French fried	20 strips	428	6.8	20	3.4	0	56	24	2.0	10	0	0.20	0.12	4.8	32
Tomato sauce (catsup)	1 tbsp.	16	0.3	0	0.0	0	4	3	0.1	156	105	0.01	0.01	0.2	2
Apple/raw	1 med	80	0.3	1	0.0	0	20	10	0.4	1	120	0.04	0.03	0.1	6
Soda pop/root beer	12 oz.	140	0.0	0	0.0	0	36	17	0.2	45	0	0.00	0.00	0.0	0
Coleslaw	1 c	173	1.6	17	1.0	5	6	53	0.5	144	190	0.06	0.06	0.4	35
Spaghetti/meat balls/sauce	1 c	332	18.6	12	3.0	75	39	124	3.7	1,009	1,590	0.25	0.30	4.0	22
Pie/apple	1 pc. (3.5 in.)	302	2.6	13	3.5	120	45	9	0.4	355	40	0.02	0.02	0.5	1
Totals Day One		2,444	77.3	111	29.8	609	298	1,015	14.1	4,802	3,744	1.0	1.8	18.3	110

*Computer software available through Morton Publishing Company

FIGURE 5.7 ❖ Computerized nutrient analysis.*

	Calo- ries	Pro- tein gm	Fat %	Sat Fat %	Cho- les- terol mg	Car- bohy- drate %	Cal- cium mg	Iron mg	Sodium mg	Vit A I.U.	Thi- amin mg	Ribo- fla- vin mg	Nia- cin mg	Vit C mg
Day One	2,444	77.3	40	11	609	48	1,015	14.1	4,802	3,744	1.0	1.8	18.3	110
Day Two	2,234	105.1	44	12	536	37	639	20.6	5,719	1,902	1.1	1.7	21.6	60
Day Three	2,491	92.0	43	19	603	43	1,787	14.7	3,919	6,351	1.6	3.5	18.2	55
Three Day Average	2,390	91.5	42	14	583	43	1,147	16.5	4,813	3,999	1.3	2.3	19.4	75
RDA	1,904*	51.2	<30	<10	<300	50>	1,200	15.0	1,904	4,000	1.1	1.3	15.0	60

*Estimated caloric value based on gender, current body weight, and activity rating (does not include additional calories burned through a physical exercise program).

OBSERVATIONS

Daily caloric intake should be distributed in such a way that 50 to 60 percent of the total calories come from carbohydrates and less than 30 percent of the total calories from fat. Protein intake should be about .8 to 1.5 grams per kilogram of body weight or about 15 to 20 percent of the total calories. Pregnant women need to consume an additional 15 grams of daily protein, while lactating women should have an extra 20 grams of daily protein (these additional grams of protein are already included in the RDA values for pregnant and lactating women). Saturated fats should constitute less than 10 percent of the total daily caloric intake.
Please note that the daily listings of food intake express the amount of carbohydrates, fat, saturated fat, and protein in grams. However, on the daily analysis and the RDA, only the amount of protein is given in grams. The amount of carbohydrates, fat, and saturated fat are expressed in percent of total calories. The final percentages are based on the total grams and total calories for all days analyzed, not from the average of the daily percentages.

If your average intake for protein, fat, saturated fat, cholesterol, or sodium is high, refer to the daily listings and decrease the intake of foods that are high in those nutrients. If your diet is deficient in carbohydrates, calcium, iron, vitamin A, thiamin, riboflavin, niacin, or vitamin C, refer to the statements below and increase your intake of the indicated foods or consult the list of selected foods in your textbook.

Caloric intake may be too high.

Total fat intake is too high.

Saturated fat intake is too high, which increases your risk for coronary heart disease.

Dietary cholesterol intake is too high. An average consumption of dietary cholesterol above 300 mg/day increases the risk for coronary heart disease. Do you know your blood cholesterol level?

Carbohydrate intake is low. Good sources of carbohydrates are whole grain breads and cereals, pasta, rice, fruits, and vegetables such as potatoes and peas.

Calcium intake is low. Good sources of calcium are milk, yogurt, cheese, green leafy vegetables, dried beans, sardines, and salmon.

Sodium intake is high.

Vitamin A intake is low. Foods high in vitamin A include skim milk fortified with vit. A, cheese, butter, fortified margarine, eggs (yolk), liver, and dark green/yellow fruits and vegetables.

*Computer software available through Morton Publishing Company

FIGURE 5.7 ✤ Computerized nutrient analysis (continued).*

Weight Management

CHAPTER 6

KEY TERMS

Basal metabolic rate (BMR)

Energy-balancing equation

Obesity

Overweight

Setpoint

Tolerable weight

OBJECTIVES

✤ Learn about myths and fallacies regarding weight management.

✤ Understand the physiology of weight control.

✤ Become familiar with the effects of diet and exercise on resting metabolic rate.

✤ Recognize the role of a lifetime exercise program as the key to a successful weight management program.

✤ Learn to write and implement a sound weight control program.

✤ Learn behavior modification techniques that help a person adhere to a lifetime weight maintenance program.

Approximately 65 million Americans are either overweight or consider themselves to be overweight. Of these, 30 million are obese. About 50% of all women and 25% of all men are on diets at any given moment. People spend about $40 billion to $50 billion yearly attempting to lose weight. More than $10 billion goes to memberships in weight reduction centers and another $30 billion to diet food sales.

Achieving and maintaining ideal body weight is a major objective of a good physical fitness program. The assessment of recommended body weight was discussed in detail in Chapter 2. Next to poor cardiorespiratory fitness, obesity is the most frequently encountered problem in fitness and wellness assessments.

Two terms commonly used in reference to people who weigh more than recommended are: overweight and obese. Overweight indicates excess weight when compared to a given standard such as height or recommended percent body fat. Obesity is defined as *a chronic disease characterized by an excessively high amount of body fat in relation to lean body mass.* Obesity levels are established at a point at which the excess body fat can lead to serious health problems.

Obesity by itself has been associated with critical health problems and accounts for 15% to 20% of the annual mortality rate in the United States. Obesity is a major risk factor for diseases of the cardiovascular system, including coronary heart disease, hypertension, congestive heart failure, high levels of blood lipids, atherosclerosis, strokes, thromboembolitic disease, diabetes, osteoarthritis, varicose veins, and intermittent claudication.

Other research points toward a possible link between obesity and cancer of the colon, rectum, prostate, gallbladder, breast, uterus, and ovaries. In addition, obesity has been associated with diabetes, ruptured intervertebral discs, gallstones, gout, respiratory insufficiency, and complications during pregnancy and delivery. Furthermore, it is implicated in psychological maladjustment and a higher accidental death rate.

Overweight and obesity are not the same thing. Most overweight people (10 to 15 pounds) are not obese. The health consequences of obesity apply primarily to significantly overweight individuals.

Granted, genetic differences exist. Some moderately overweight people have health problems, but this is not the case for most. Moderately overweight people with diabetes or other cardiovascular risk factors, however, benefit from weight loss.

TOLERABLE WEIGHT

Many people want to lose weight so they will look better. That's a noteworthy goal. The problem, however, is that they often have a distorted image of what they really would look like if they were to reduce to what they think is their "ideal" weight. Hereditary factors play a big role, and only a small fraction of the population has the genes for a "perfect body." Tolerable

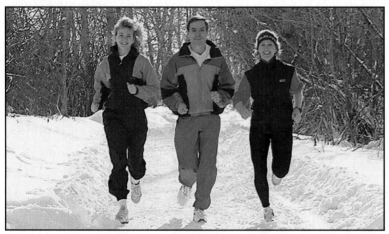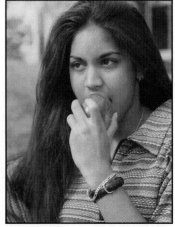

Achieving and maintaining a high physical fitness percent body fat standard requires a lifetime commitment to regular physical activity and proper nutrition.

weight is a more realistic goal. This is a realistic standard that is *not "ideal" but is acceptable*. It is likely to be closer to the health-fitness standard rather than the physical-fitness standard for many people.

As people set their own target weight, they should be realistic. Attaining the high physical fitness percent body fat standard in Table 2.10, Chapter 2, is extremely difficult for some people. This standard is even more difficult to maintain, unless they are willing to make a commitment to a *vigorous* lifetime exercise program and permanent dietary changes. Few people are willing to do that. The health-fitness percent body fat category may be more realistic for these people.

A question you should ask yourself is: Are you happy with your weight? Part of enjoying a better quality of life is being happy with yourself. If you are not, you either should do something about it or learn to live with it!

If you are above the health-fitness percent body fat standard, you should try to come down and stay there, for health reasons. This is the percent body fat at which there seems to be no detriment to health.

If you have achieved the health-fitness standard but would like to be better, you need to ask yourself a second question: How badly do I want it? Do you want it enough to implement lifetime exercise and dietary changes? If you are not willing to change, you should stop worrying about your weight and deem the health-fitness standard as tolerable for you.

PRINCIPLES OF WEIGHT MANAGEMENT

The energy-balancing equation states that *when caloric intake equals caloric output, weight remains unchanged*. If caloric input exceeds output, the person gains weight. When caloric output is more than intake, the individual loses weight.

Each pound of fat equals 3,500 calories. Therefore, theoretically, to increase body fat (weight) by 1 pound, a person would have to consume an excess of 3,500 calories. Equally, to lose 1 pound, the individual would have to decrease caloric intake by 3,500 calories. This principle seems straight-forward, but, as you will learn later in this chapter, it is not quite that simple with the human body.

Only about 10% of all people who begin a traditional weight-loss program (without exercise) are able to lose the desired weight. Worse, less than 1% of this group is able to keep the weight off for a significant time. Traditional diets have failed because few of them incorporate lifetime changes in food selection and exercise as the keys to successful weight loss and maintenance. Yet, fad diets continue to deceive people, and promoters claim that the dieter will lose weight by following all the instructions.

Most diets are low in calories and deprive the body of certain nutrients, generating a metabolic imbalance that can even cause death. Under these conditions, a lot of the weight lost is in the form of water and protein, not fat.

Overly fat individuals who go on a crash diet lose nearly half the weight in lean (protein) tissue[1] (see Figure 6.1). When the body uses protein instead of a combination of fats and carbohydrates as a source of energy, weight is lost as much as 10 times faster.[2] A gram of protein produces half the amount of energy that fat does. In the case of muscle protein, one-fifth of protein is mixed with four-fifths of water. Each pound of muscle yields only one-tenth the amount of energy as a pound of fat. As a result, most of the weight loss is in the form of water, which on the scale, of course, looks good.

Some diets allow only certain specialized foods. If people would realize that no "magic" foods provide all the necessary nutrients, and that a person has to eat a variety of foods to be well-nourished, the diet industry would not be as successful. Most of these diets create a nutritional deficiency, which at times are fatal. The reason some of these diets succeed is that people eventually get tired of eating the same thing day in and day out and start eating less. If they achieve the lower weight without making permanent

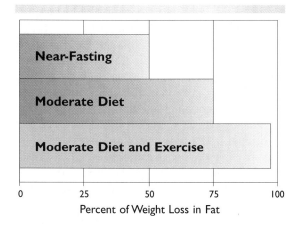

Adapted from *Alive Man: The Physiology of Physical Activity*, by R. J. Shephard (Springfield, IL: Charles C Thomas, 1975), p. 484–488.

FIGURE 6.1 ♣ Effects of three forms of diet on fat loss.

dietary changes, however, they quickly gain back the weight once they go back to old eating habits.

A few diets recommend exercise along with caloric restrictions — the best method for weight reduction, of course. A lot of the weight lost is because of the exercise, so the diet achieves its purpose. As discussed later in this chapter, exercise in itself plays a major role in how much a person weighs. Unfortunately, if people do not permanently change their food selection and activity level, they gain back the weight quickly after discontinuing dieting and exercise.

Only a few years ago the principles governing a weight loss and maintenance program seemed to be fairly clear, but we now know the final answers are not in yet. Traditional concepts related to weight control have centered on three assumptions:

1. Balancing food intake against output allows a person to achieve recommended weight.

2. Fat people just eat too much.

3. The human body doesn't care how much (or little) fat is stored.

Although these statements may contain some truth, they are still open to much debate and research.

Every person has a *unique body fat percentage regulated by genetic and environmental factors*, referred to as setpoint or the *fat thermostat*. The genetic instinct to survive tells the body that fat storage is vital, and, therefore, the setpoint sets an acceptable fat level. This setpoint remains somewhat constant or may climb gradually because of poor lifestyle habits.

Especially under strict calorie reduction (fewer than 800 calories per day), the body makes compensatory metabolic adjustments in an effort to maintain its fat storage. The basal metabolic rate (BMR), the *lowest level of oxygen consumption necessary to sustain life*, may drop dramatically against a consistent negative caloric balance, and a person may be on a plateau for days or even weeks without losing much weight. When the dieter goes back to the normal or even below-normal caloric intake, at which the weight may have been stable for a long time, he or she quickly regains the fat loss as the body strives to regain a comfortable fat store.

These findings were substantiated by research conducted at Rockefeller University in New York.[3] The authors showed that the body resists maintenance of altered weight. Obese and lifetime nonobese individuals were used in the investigation. Following a 10% weight loss, in an attempt to regain the lost weight, the body compensated by burning up to 15% fewer calories than expected for the new reduced weight (after accounting for the 10% loss). The effects were similar in the obese and nonobese participants. These results imply that after a 10% weight loss, a person would have to eat less or exercise more to account for the estimated deficit of about 200 to 300 daily calories.

In this same study, when the participants were allowed to increase their weight to 10% above their "normal" body weight (pre-weight loss), the body burned 10% to 15% more calories than expected. This indicates an attempt by the body to waste energy and return to the preset weight. The study provides another indication that the body is highly resistant to weight changes unless additional lifestyle changes are incorporated to ensure successful weight management. Methods to manage weight will be discussed in this chapter.

This research shows why most dieters regain weight lost through dietary means alone. Let's use a practical illustration: Jim would like to lose some body fat and assumes that he has reached a stable body weight at an average daily caloric intake of 2,500 calories (no weight gain or loss at this daily intake). In an attempt to lose weight rapidly, he now goes on a strict low-calorie diet (or, even worse, a near-fasting diet). Immediately the body activates its survival mechanism and readjusts its metabolism to a lower caloric balance.

After a few weeks of dieting at under 400 to 600 calories per day, the body now can maintain its normal functions at 1,000 calories per day. Having lost the desired weight, he terminates the diet but realizes the original intake of 2,500 calories per day will have to be lower to maintain the new lower weight.

To adjust to the new lower body weight, the intake is restricted to about 2,200 calories per day. Jim is surprised to find that even at this lower daily intake (300 fewer calories), weight comes back at a rate of about one pound every one to two weeks. After the diet ends, this new lowered metabolic rate may take several months to kick back up to its normal level.

From this explanation, individuals clearly should never go on very low-calorie diets. Not only will this decrease the resting metabolic rate, but it also will deprive the body of basic daily nutrients required for normal function. Under no circumstances should a person go on a diet that calls for below 1,200 and 1,500 calories for women and men, respectively. Weight (fat) is gained over months and years, not overnight. Equally, weight loss should be gradual, not abrupt. A daily caloric intake of 1,200 to 1,500 calories provides the necessary nutrients if properly distributed over the various food groups (meeting the minimum daily required servings

from each group). Of course, the individual has to learn which foods meet the requirements and yet are low in fat, sugar, and calories.

Furthermore, when a person tries to lose weight by dietary restrictions alone, lean body mass (muscle protein, along with vital organ protein) always decreases. The amount of lean body mass lost depends entirely on caloric limitation. When obese people go on a near-fasting diet, up to half of the weight loss can be lean body mass and the other half, actual fat loss. When the diet is combined with exercise, close to 100% of the weight loss is in the form of fat, and lean tissue actually may increase (see Figure 6.1). Loss of lean body mass is never good because it weakens the organs and muscles and slows down the metabolism.

Reductions in lean body mass are common in people who are on severely restricted diets. No diet with caloric intakes below 1,200 to 1,500 calories will prevent loss of lean body mass. Even at this intake level, some loss is inevitable unless the diet is combined with exercise. Many diets claim they do not alter the lean component, but the simple truth is that, regardless of what nutrients may be added to the diet, caloric restrictions always prompt a loss of lean tissue.

Too many people go on low-calorie diets again and again. Every time they do, the metabolic rate slows down as more lean tissue is lost. Many people in their 40s or older who weigh the same as they did when they were 20 think they are at recommended body weight. During this span of 20 years or more, they may have dieted too many times without exercising. They regain the weight shortly after terminating each diet, but most of that gain is in fat. Maybe at age 20 they weighed 150 pounds, of which only 15% to 16% was fat. Now at age 40, even though they still weigh 150 pounds, they might be 30% fat (see Figure 6.2 and also Figure 2.1 in Chapter 2). At recommended body weight, they wonder why they are eating so little and still having trouble staying at that weight.

Further, a diet high in fats and refined carbohydrates, near-fasting diets, and perhaps even artificial sweeteners keep people from losing

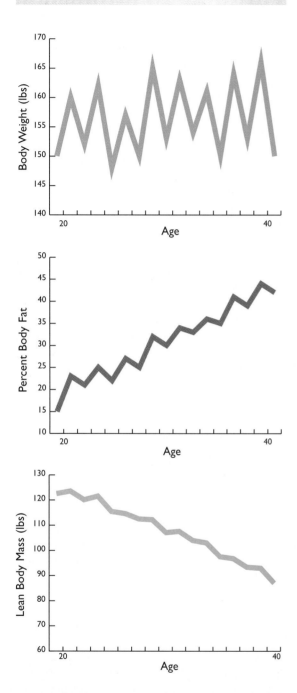

FIGURE 6.2 ❖ Effects of frequent dieting without exercise on body weight, percent body fat, and lean body mass.

weight successfully. To the contrary, these practices contribute to fat gain. *The only practical and sensible way to lose fat weight is by combining exercise and a sensible diet high in complex carbohydrates and low in fat and sugar.*

After studying the effects of proper food management, many nutritionists now believe the source of calories should be the primary concern in a weight-control program. Most of the effort in this regard is spent in retraining eating habits, increasing the intake of complex carbohydrates and high-fiber foods, and decreasing the consumption of refined carbohydrates (sugars) and fats. For most people, this change in eating habits brings about a decrease in total daily caloric intake.

A "diet" is no longer viewed as a temporary tool to aid in weight loss but, instead, as a permanent change in eating behaviors to ensure weight management and better health. The role of increased physical activity also must be considered because successful weight loss, and recommended body composition seldom are attainable without a moderate reduction in caloric intake combined with a regular exercise program.

EXERCISE: THE KEY TO SUCCESSFUL WEIGHT MANAGEMENT

A more effective way to tilt the energy balancing equation in your favor is by burning calories through physical activity. Exercise also seems to exert control over how much a person weighs.

If, starting at age 25, the typical American gains 1 pound of weight per year, this represents a simple energy surplus of under 10 calories per day (10 × 365 = 3,650). In most cases the additional weight accumulated in middle age comes from people becoming less physically active and not as a result of increasing caloric intake. Dr. Jack Wilmore, a leading exercise physiologist and expert weight management researcher, stated:[4]

> Physical inactivity is certainly a major, if not the primary, cause of obesity in the United

States today. A certain minimal level of activity might be necessary for us to accurately balance our caloric intake to our caloric expenditure. With too little activity, we appear to lose the fine control we normally have to maintain this incredible balance. This fine balance amounts to less than 10 calories per day, or the equivalent of one potato chip.

If a person is trying to lose weight, a combination of aerobic and strength-training exercises works best. Because of the continuity and duration of aerobic exercise, it burns many calories. Strength training, on the other hand, has the greatest impact on increasing lean body mass.

The role of aerobic exercise in successful lifetime weight management cannot be underestimated. As illustrated in Figure 6.3, greater

weight loss is achieved by combining a diet with an aerobic exercise program.[5] Of even greater significance, only the individuals who participated in an 18-month post-diet aerobic exercise program were able to keep off the weight. Those who discontinued exercise gained weight. Furthermore, all those who initiated or resumed exercise during the 18-month follow-up were able to lose weight again. Individuals who only dieted and never exercised regained 60% and 92% of their weight loss at the 6- and 18-month follow-ups, respectively.

Faster weight loss can be obtained by combining aerobic exercise with a strength-training program. Two exercise groups, a 30-minute aerobic group and a 15-minute aerobic plus 15-minute strength-training (30 minutes total) group participated in an 8-week, 3-days-per-week study. Both groups followed a dietary plan that consisted of approximately 60% carbohydrates, 20% fats, and 20% proteins.

Results of the investigation[6] showed that the aerobic group lost an average of 3½ pounds, 3

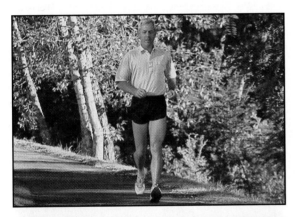

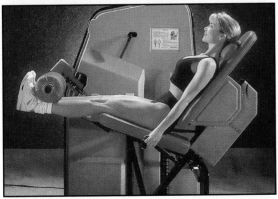

Regular participation in a combined lifetime aerobic and strength-training exercise program is the key to successful weight management.

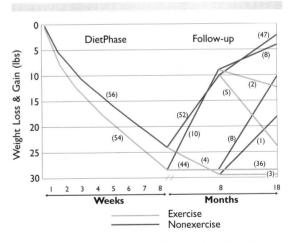

Note: Numbers in parentheses indicate number of participants.

Source: "Exercise as an Adjunct to Weight Loss and Maintenance in Moderately Obese Subjects," *American Journal of Clinical Nutrition,* 49 (1989), 115–1123.

FIGURE 6.3 ❖ Aerobic exercise and weight loss and maintenance in moderately obese individuals.

of which were fat, and the remaining ½ pound was lean tissue. The combined aerobic and strength-training group lost an average of 8 pounds. Changes in body composition, however, indicated that the latter group actually lost 10 pounds of fat and gained 2 pounds of lean tissue (see Figure 6.4). These findings indicate that a sensible strength training program helps in losing weight and maintaining muscle mass and metabolic rate.

Another point of interest is that each additional pound of muscle tissue can raise the basal metabolic rate by 35 calories per day.[7] Thus, an individual who adds 5 pounds of muscle tissue as a result of strength training increases the basal metabolic rate by 175 calories per day (35 × 5), which equals 63,875 calories per year (175 × 365), or the equivalent of 18.25 pounds of fat (63,875 ÷ 3,500).

Because exercise promotes an increase in lean body mass, body weight often remains the same or even increases after beginning an exercise program, while inches and percent body fat decrease. More lean tissue means more functional capacity of the human body. With exercise, most of the weight loss becomes apparent after a few weeks of training, when the lean component has stabilized.

Research has revealed the fallacy of spot reducing or losing cellulite, as some people call the fat deposits that bulge out in certain areas of the body. These deposits are nothing but enlarged fat cells from accumulated body fat. *Merely doing several sets of sit-ups daily will not get rid of fat in the midsection of the body.* When fat comes off, it does so throughout the entire body, not just the exercised area. The greatest proportion of fat may come off the biggest fat deposits, but the caloric output of a few sets of sit-ups has almost no effect on reducing total body fat. A person has to exercise much longer to really see results.

Dieting never has been fun and never will be. People who are overweight and are serious about losing weight will have to make exercise a regular part of their daily life, along with proper food management and perhaps a sensible cut in

caloric intake. Some precautions are in order, as excessive body fat is a risk factor for cardiovascular disease. Depending on the extent of the weight problem, a medical examination and possibly a stress ECG may be necessary before undertaking the exercise program. A physician should be consulted in this regard.

Significantly overweight individuals also may have to choose activities in which they will not have to support their own body weight but still will be effective in burning calories. Joint and muscle injuries are common in overweight individuals who participate in weight-bearing exercises such as walking, jogging, and aerobics.

Better alternatives for overweight people are riding a bicycle (either road or stationary), water aerobics, walking in a shallow pool, or running in place in deep water (treading water). The last three modes of exercise are quickly gaining in popularity because little skill is required for participation. These activities seem to be just as effective as other forms of aerobic activity in helping individuals lose weight without the pain and the fear of injuries.

One final benefit of exercise for weight control is that it allows fat to be burned more efficiently. Both carbohydrates and fats are sources of energy. When the glucose levels begin to drop

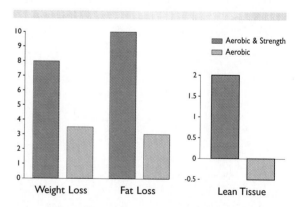

Source: "You Can Sell Exercise for Weight Loss," by W. L. Wescott, *Fitness Management*, 7:12 (1991), 33–34.

FIGURE 6.4 ✤ Changes in body composition through an aerobic exercise program and a combined aerobic/strength-training exercise program.

TABLE 6.2 ✤ Caloric Expenditure of Selected Physical Activities

Activity*	Cal/lb/min**	Activity*	Cal/lb/min**	Activity*	Cal/lb/min**
Aerobelt Exercise		Dance		StairMaster	
Aero-belt Jogging/		Moderate	0.030	Moderate	0.070
6 mph	0.098	Vigorous	0.055	Vigorous	0.090
Aero-belt		Golf	0.030	Stationary Cycling	
Step-Aerobics/8"	0.105	Gymnastics		Moderate	0.055
Aero-belt Walking/		Light	0.030	Vigorous	0.070
4 mph	0.073	Heavy	0.056	Strength Training	0.050
Aerobics		Handball	0.064	Swimming (crawl)	
Moderate	0.065	Hiking	0.040	20 yds/min	0.031
High Impact	0.095	Judo/Karate	0.086	25 yds/min	0.040
Step-Aerobics	0.070	Racquetball	0.065	45 yds/min	0.057
Archery	0.030	Rope Jumping	0.060	50 yds/min	0.070
Badminton		Rowing (vigorous)	0.090	Table Tennis	0.030
Recreation	0.038	Running		Tennis	
Competition	0.065	11.0 min/mile	0.070	Moderate	0.045
Baseball	0.031	8.5 min/mile	0.090	Competition	0.064
Basketball		7.0 min/mile	0.102	Volleyball	0.030
Moderate	0.046	6.0 min/mile	0.114	Walking	
Competition	0.063	Deep water***	0.100	4.5 mph	0.045
Bowling	0.030	Skating (moderate)	0.038	Shallow pool	0.090
Calisthenics	0.033	Skiing		Water Aerobics	
Cycling (level)		Downhill	0.060	Moderate	0.050
5.5 mph	0.033	Level (5 mph)	0.078	Vigorous	0.070
10.0 mph	0.050	Soccer	0.059	Wrestling	0.085
13.0 mph	0.071				

*Values are only for actual time engaged in the activity.

**Cal/lb/min = calories per pound of body weight per minute of activity

***Treading water

Adapted from *Fitness for Life: An Individualized Approach,* by P. E. Allsen, J. M. Harrison, and B. Vance (Dubuque, IA: Wm. C. Brown, 1989); *Fitness for College and Life,* by C. A. Bucher, and W. E. Prentice (St. Louis: Times Mirror/Mosby College Publishing, 1989); *Physiological Measurements of Metabolic Functions in Man,* by C. F. Consolazio, R. E. Johnson, and L. J. Pecora (New York: McGraw-Hill, 1963); *Physical Fitness: The Pathway to Healthful Living,* by R. V. Hockey (St. Louis: Times Mirror/Mosby College Publishing, 1989); and research conducted at Boise State University by W. W. K. Hoeger et al, 1986–1993.

on a diet, weight is lost most effectively if he or she consumes most of the calories before 1:00 p.m. and not during the evening meal. This center recommends that when a person is attempting to lose weight, intake should consist of a minimum of 25% of the total daily calories for breakfast, 50% for lunch, and 25% or less at dinner.

Other experts have reported that if most of the daily calories are consumed during one meal, the body may perceive that something is wrong and will slow down the metabolism so it can store a greater amount of calories in the form of fat. Also, eating most of the calories in one meal causes a person to go hungry the rest of the day, making it harder to adhere to the diet.

TIPS FOR A LIFETIME WEIGHT MANAGEMENT PROGRAM

Achieving and maintaining recommended body composition is by no means impossible, but it does require desire and commitment. If adequate weight management is to become a reality, some retraining of behavior is crucial for success. Modifying old habits and developing new, positive behaviors take time. Individuals have applied the following management techniques to change detrimental behavior successfully and adhere to a positive lifetime weight control program. In developing a retraining program, people are not expected to use all of the strategies listed but should pick the ones that apply to them.

1. *Have a commitment to change.* The first necessary ingredient to modify behavior is the desire to do so. The reasons for change must be more compelling than those for continuing present lifestyle patterns. You must accept that you have a problem and decide by yourself whether you really want to change. If you are sincerely committed, the chances for success are enhanced already.

2. *Set realistic goals.* Most people with a weight problem would like to lose weight in a relatively short time but fail to realize that the weight problem developed over a span of several years. A sound weight reduction and maintenance program can be accomplished only by establishing new lifetime eating and exercise habits, both of which take time to develop.

   In setting a realistic long-term goal, short-term objectives also should be planned. The long-term goal may be to decrease body fat to 20% of total body weight. The short-term objective may be a 1% decrease in body fat each month. Objectives like these allow for regular evaluation and help maintain motivation and renewed commitment to attain the long-term goal.

3. *Incorporate exercise into the program.* Choosing enjoyable activities, places, times, equipment, and people to work with helps a person adhere to an exercise program. Details on developing a complete exercise program are given in Chapter 3.

4. *Develop healthy eating patterns.* Plan on eating three regular meals per day consistent with the body's nutritional requirements, and learn to differentiate hunger from appetite. Hunger is the actual physical need for food. Appetite is a desire for food, usually triggered by factors such as stress, habit, boredom, depression, food availability, or just the thought of food itself. Individuals should eat only when they have a physical need. In this regard, developing and sticking to a regular meal pattern help control hunger.

5. *Avoid automatic eating.* Many people associate certain daily activities with eating. For example, people eat while cooking, watching television, reading, talking on the telephone, or visiting with neighbors. Most of the time, the foods consumed in these situations lack nutritional value or are high in sugar and fat.

6. *Stay busy.* People tend to eat more when they sit around and do nothing. Occupying the mind and body with activities not associated with eating helps take away the desire to eat. Walking, cycling, playing sports, gardening, sewing, or visiting a library, a museum, a park are some options. People might develop other skills and interests or try something new and exciting to break the routine of life.

7. *Plan meals ahead of time.* Sensible shopping is essential to accomplish this objective. (By the way, shop on a full stomach, because hungry shoppers tend to buy unhealthy foods impulsively — and then snack on the way home). The shopping list should include whole-grain breads and cereals, fruits and vegetables, low-fat milk and dairy products, lean meats, fish, and poultry.

8. *Cook wisely.*
   - ❖ Use less fat and refined foods in food preparation.
   - ❖ Trim all visible fat from meats and remove skin from poultry before cooking.
   - ❖ Skim the fat off gravies and soups.
   - ❖ Bake, broil, and boil instead of frying.
   - ❖ Sparingly use butter, cream, mayonnaise, and salad dressings.
   - ❖ Avoid coconut oil, palm oil, and cocoa butter.
   - ❖ Prepare plenty of bulky foods.
   - ❖ Add whole-grain breads and cereals, vegetables, and legumes to most meals.
   - ❖ Try fruits for dessert.
   - ❖ Beware of soda pop, fruit juices, and fruit-flavored drinks.
   - ❖ In addition to sugar, cut down on other refined carbohydrates such as corn syrup, malt sugar, dextrose, and fructose.
   - ❖ Drink plenty of water — at least six glasses a day.

9. *Do not serve more food than you should eat.* Measure the food in portions, and keep serving dishes away from the table. This means you will eat less, have a harder time getting seconds, and have less appetite because the food is not visible. People should not be forced to eat when they are satisfied (including children after they already have had a healthy, nutritious serving).

10. *Eat slowly and at the table only.* Eating is one of the pleasures of life, and we need to take time to enjoy it. Eating on the run is not good because the body doesn't have enough time to "register" nutritive and caloric consumption and people overeat before the body perceives the fullness signal. Always eating at the table also forces people to take time out to eat, and it deters snacking between meals, primarily because of the extra time and effort required to sit down and eat. When people are done eating, they should not sit around the table but, rather, clean up and put away the food to keep from unnecessary snacking.

11. *Avoid social binges.* Social gatherings tend to entice self-defeating behavior. Visual imagery might help before attending any social gatherings: Plan ahead and visualize yourself in that gathering. Do not feel pressured to eat or drink, and don't rationalize in these situations. Choose low-calorie foods, and entertain yourself with other activities such as dancing and talking.

12. *Do not raid the refrigerator and the cookie jar.* In these tempting situations take control. Stop and think what is happening. Environmental management is another tactic: Do not bring high-calorie, high-sugar, or high-fat foods into the house. If they are there already, store them where they are hard to get to or see. If they are out of sight or not readily available, the temptation is less. Keeping food in places such as the garage and basement tends to discourage people from taking the time and effort to get them. By no means should you have to eliminate treats entirely, but all things should be done in moderation.

13. *Practice stress-management techniques.* Many people snack and increase food consumption in stressful situations. Eating is not a stress-releasing activity and instead can aggravate the problem if weight control is an issue.

14. *Monitor changes and reward accomplishments.* Feedback on fat loss and lean tissue gain is a reward in itself. Awareness of changes in body composition also helps reinforce new behaviors. Being able to exercise without interruption for 15, 20, 30, 60 minutes, swimming a certain distance, running a mile — all these accomplishments deserve recognition. Meeting objectives calls for rewards but not related to eating — new clothing, a tennis racquet, a bicycle, exercise shoes, or something else that is

special and you would not have acquired otherwise.

15. *Think positive.* Negative thoughts about how difficult changing past behaviors might be, are detracting. It's better to think of the benefits you will reap, such as feeling, looking, and functioning better, plus enjoying better health and improving the quality of life. Avoid negative environments and people who will not be supportive.

IN CONCLUSION

There is no simple and quick way to take off excessive body fat and keep it off for good.

Weight management is accomplished through a lifetime commitment to physical activity and proper food selection. When taking part in a weight (fat) reduction program, people have to decrease their caloric intake moderately and implement strategies to modify unhealthy eating behaviors.

During the process of behavior modification, relapses into past negative behaviors are almost inevitable. Making mistakes is human and does not necessarily mean failure. Failure comes to those who give up and do not use previous experiences to build upon and, instead, develop skills that will prevent self-defeating behaviors in the future. "Where there's a will, there's a way," and those who persist will reap the rewards.

NOTES

1. R. J. Shepard, *Alive Man: The Physiology of Physical Activity* (Springfield, IL: Charles C Thomas, 1975), pp. 484–488

2. D. Remington, A. G. Fisher, and E. A. Parent, *How to Lower Your Fat Thermostat* (Provo, UT: Vitality House International, 1983).

3. R. L. Leibel, M. Rosenbaum, and J. Hirsh, "Changes in Energy Expenditure Resulting from Altered Body Weight," *New England Journal of Medicine*, 332(1995), 621–628.

4. J. H. Wilmore. "Exercise, Obesity, and Weight Control," *Physical Activity and Fitness Research Digest.* (Washington DC: President's Council on Physical Fitness & Sports, 1994).

5. K. N. Pavlou, S. Krey, and W. P. Steffe, "Exercise as an Adjunct to Weight Loss and Maintenance in Moderately Obese Subjects," *American Journal of Clinical Nutrition*, 49 (1989), 1115–1123.

6. W. L. Wescott. "You Can Sell Exercise for Weight Loss." *Fitness Management*, 7:12 (1991), 33–34.

7. W. W. Campbell, M. C. Crim, V. R. Young, and W. J. Evans, "Increased Energy Requirements and Changes in Body Composition with Resistance Training in Older Adults," *American Journal of Clinical Nutrition*, 60 (1994), 167–175.

A Healthy Lifestyle Approach

KEY TERMS

Acquired immunodeficiency syndrome (AIDS)

Altruism

Angiogenesis

Atherosclerosis

Benign

Blood lipids

Blood pressure

Breathing techniques

Cancer

Carcinoma in situ

Cardiovascular diseases

Cholesterol

Chronic obstructive pulmonary disease (COPD)

Chronological age

Coronary heart disease (CHD)

Cruciferous vegetables

Deoxyribonucleic acid (DNA)

Diabetes mellitus

Electrocardiogram (ECG or EKG)

Exercise ECG

Fight-or-flight mechanism

Functional age

HDL-cholesterol

Human immuno-deficiency virus (HIV)

Hypertension

LDL-cholesterol

Malignant

Metastasis

Nonmelanoma skin cancer

Progressive muscle relaxation

Risk factors

Sexually transmitted diseases (STDs)

Spirituality

Stress

Triglycerides

Very low-density lipoproteins (VLDLs)

OBJECTIVES

❖ Learn the importance of implementing a healthy lifestyle program.

❖ Understand the major risk factors for coronary heart disease.

❖ Become acquainted with cancer-prevention guidelines.

❖ Learn how to cope with stress.

❖ Recognize the relationship between spirituality and wellness.

❖ Learn the health consequences of chemical abuse and irresponsible sex.

*A*lthough people in the United States believe firmly in the benefits of physical activity and positive lifestyle habits as means to promote better health, most do not reap these benefits because they simply do not know how to put into practice a sound fitness and wellness program that will lead to a higher quality of life. Further, the present lifestyle of many Americans is such a serious threat to their health that it actually leads to premature illness and mortality. Improving the quality, and most likely the lengthy, of our lives is a matter of personal choice. Experts term the combination of a fitness program and a healthy lifestyle program the "wellness approach" to better health and quality of life.

As defined in Chapter 1, wellness is the constant and deliberate effort to stay healthy and achieve the highest potential for well-being. Wellness incorporates healthy lifestyle factors such as good fitness and nutrition, stress management, disease prevention, social support and self-worth, spirituality, substance abuse control, personal safety, and health education (see Figure 7.1).

The difference between physical fitness and wellness is best illustrated in the following example. An individual who runs 3 miles a day, lifts weights regularly, participates in stretching exercises, and controls his or her body weight can easily be classified in the high physical fitness category for each of the fitness components. If this same individual, however, has high blood pressure, smokes, is under constant stress, consumes too much alcohol, and eats too many fatty foods, he or she probably is developing several risk factors for disease and may not be aware of it. Risk factors are *lifestyle and genetic components that may lead to disease.*

Consequently, our biggest challenge at the end of this century is to learn how to take control of our personal health habits by engaging in positive lifestyle activities. To help you determine how your lifestyle habits are contributing to your health, the National Health Information Clearinghouse developed a simple healthstyle self-test, contained in Appendix F. Researchers also point out 10 simple lifestyle habits that can increase longevity significantly:

1. Participate in a lifetime exercise program.
2. Do not smoke cigarettes.
3. Eat a balanced diet.
4. Maintain recommended body weight.
5. Sleep 7 to 8 hours each night.
6. Decrease stress levels.
7. Drink alcohol moderately or not at all.
8. Surround yourself with healthy relationships.
9. Be informed about the environment and avoid environmental risk factors.
10. Take personal safety measures.

MAJOR HEALTH PROBLEMS IN THE UNITED STATES

Of all deaths in the United States, 66% are caused by cardiovascular disease and cancer.[1] Close to 80% of these deaths could be prevented by a healthy lifestyle program. The third and fourth leading causes of death, chronic and obstructive pulmonary disease and accidents, also are preventable, primarily by abstaining from tobacco and other drugs, wearing seat belts, and using common sense.

In looking at the underlying causes of death in the United States, estimates[2] (see Figure 7.2) indicate that 9 of the 10 causes are related to lifestyle and lack of common sense. The "big three" — tobacco use, poor diet and inactivity, and alcohol abuse — are responsible for more than 800,000 annual deaths.

FIGURE 7.1 ❖ Wellness components.

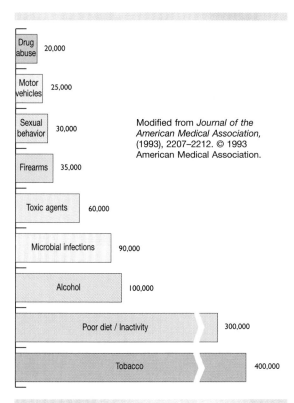

Modified from *Journal of the American Medical Association,* (1993), 2207–2212. © 1993 American Medical Association.

FIGURE 7.2 ❖ Underlying causes of death in the United States.

CARDIOVASCULAR DISEASES

The most prevalent degenerative conditions in the United States are cardiovascular diseases, those that *affect the heart and the circulatory system.* One in six men and one in eight women age 45 and older have had a heart attack or stroke.[3] Based on 1992 vital statistics, 42% of all deaths in the United States were attributable to heart and blood vessel disease.[4] Some examples of cardiovascular diseases are coronary heart disease, peripheral vascular disease, congenital heart disease, rheumatic heart disease, atherosclerosis, strokes, high blood pressure, and congestive heart failure. Table 7.1 provides the estimated prevalence and annual number of

deaths caused by the major types of cardiovascular disease.

According to the American Heart Association, the estimated cost of heart and blood vessel disease in the United States exceeded $135 billion in 1994. More than 1.5 million people have heart attacks each year, and over half a million of them die as a result. About half the time the first symptom of coronary heart disease is the heart attack itself. In one of every five cardiovascular deaths, sudden death is the initial symptom. About half of those who die are men in their most productive years of life — between ages 40 and 65.

Although heart and blood vessel disease is still the number-one health problem in the United States, the incidence has declined by 36% in the last two decades (see Figure 7.3). The main reason for this dramatic decrease is health education. More people now are aware of the risk factors for cardiovascular disease and are changing their lifestyle to lower their potential risk for this disease.

The heart and the coronary arteries are illustrated in Figure 7.4. The major form of cardiovascular disease is coronary heart disease (CHD). Heart attack, angina pectoris, and sudden

TABLE 7.1 ❖ Estimated Prevalence and Yearly Number of Deaths from Cardiovascular Disease in United States, 1992

	Prevalence	Deaths
Major forms of cardiovascular diseases*	58,920,000	925,079
Coronary heart disease	11,200,000**	
Heart attack	1,500,000	480,170
Stroke	3,080,000	143,640
High blood pressure	50,000,000	35,830
Rheumatic heart disease	1,350,000	5,960

*Includes people with one or more forms of cardiovascular disease.

**Number of deaths included under heart attack.

Source: American Heart Association, *Heart and Stroke Facts: 1995* (Statistical Supplement) (Dallas: AHA, 1994).

cardiac death are all included under CHD. In CHD the *arteries that supply the heart muscle with oxygen and nutrients are narrowed by fatty deposits* such as cholesterol and triglycerides. Narrowing of the coronary arteries diminishes the blood supply to the heart muscle, which can precipitate a heart attack. CHD is the single leading cause of death in the United States, accounting for approximately a third of all deaths and more than half of all cardiovascular deaths.

The leading contributors to the development of CHD are:

❖ Physical inactivity

❖ Low HDL-cholesterol

❖ Elevated LDL-cholesterol

❖ Smoking

❖ High blood pressure

❖ Abnormal electrocardiograms (ECG)

❖ Personal and family history of cardiovascular disease

❖ Diabetes

❖ Excessive body fat

❖ Elevated triglycerides

❖ Tension and stress

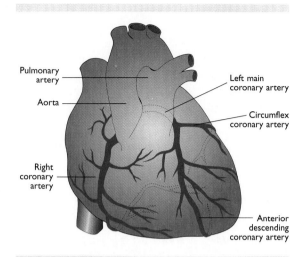

FIGURE 7.4 ❖ The heart and its blood vessels.

❖ Gender

❖ Age

An important concept in CHD risk management is that, with the exception of age, gender, family history of heart disease, and certain electrocardiographic abnormalities, all other risk factors are preventable and reversible. Individuals can control them by modifying their lifestyle. Approximately 90% of CHD is preventable if people practice healthy lifestyle habits.[5] To aid in implementing a lifetime risk reduction program, the risk factors described next should be considered.

Physical Inactivity

Improving cardiorespiratory endurance through aerobic exercise has perhaps the greatest impact in reducing the overall risk for cardiovascular disease. In this day and age of "mechanized societies," we cannot afford not to exercise. Research data on the benefits of aerobic exercise in reducing cardiovascular disease is too impressive to be ignored.

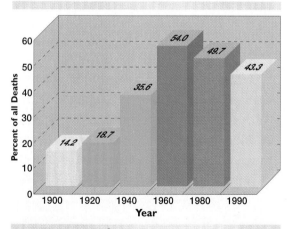

FIGURE 7.3 ❖ Incidence of cardiovascular disease in the United States for selected years: 1900–1990.

Fitness & Wellness

The guidelines for implementing an aerobic exercise program are discussed thoroughly in Chapter 3. These guidelines are ideal for developing proper cardiorespiratory fitness, enhancing health, and extending the lifespan. Even moderate amounts of aerobic exercise, however, can reduce cardiovascular risk considerably. As shown in Figure 7.5, work conducted at the Aerobics Research Institute in Dallas, Texas showed a much higher incidence of cardiovascular deaths in unfit people (group 1 in Figure 7.5) as compared to moderately fit people (groups 2 and 3).[6]

A regular aerobic exercise program helps to control most of the major risk factors that lead to heart and blood vessel disease. Aerobic exercise will:

— increase cardiorespiratory endurance.

— decrease and control blood pressure.

— reduce body fat.

— lower blood lipids (cholesterol and triglycerides).

— improve HDL-cholesterol (see later discussion).

— help control or decrease the risk for diabetes.

— increase and maintain good heart function, sometimes improving certain ECG abnormalities.

— motivate toward smoking cessation.

— alleviate tension and stress.

— counteract a personal history of heart disease.

The significance of physical inactivity in contributing to cardiovascular risk was shown clearly in 1992 when the American Heart Association added physical inactivity as one of the four major risk factors for cardiovascular disease. The other three are smoking, a poor cholesterol profile, and high blood pressure.

High Blood Pressure

Blood pressure is the *force of the blood exerted against artery walls*. Blood pressure should be checked regularly, regardless of whether it is or is not elevated. The pressure is measured in milliliters of mercury (mm Hg) and usually expressed in two numbers. The higher number reflects the *systolic pressure*, the pressure exerted during the forceful contraction of the heart. The lower value, *diastolic pressure*, is taken during the heart's relaxation phase, when no blood is being ejected.

Ideal blood pressure is 120/80 or below. The American Heart Association considers all *blood pressures over 140/90* as hypertension. Regular aerobic exercise, weight control, a low-salt/low-fat diet, smoking cessation, and stress management are the keys to blood pressure control. If needed, medications are used to lower high blood pressure.

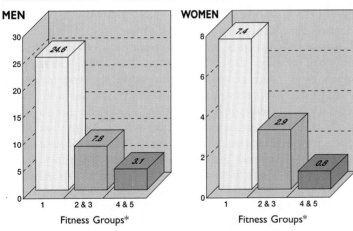

Note: Age-adjusted death rates per 10,000 person-years of follow-up, 1978–1985

From "Physical Fitness and All-Cause Mortality: A Prospective Study of Healthy Man and Woman" by S. N. Blair, H. W. Kohl, III, R. S. Paffenbarger, Jr., D. B. Clark, D. H. Cooper, and L. W. Gibbons, *Journal of the American Medical Association,* 262 (1985), 2395–2401.

FIGURE 7.5 ✤ Relationship between fitness levels and cardiovascular mortality (1970–1985).

Body Composition

As discussed in Chapter 2, body composition is the ratio of lean body weight to fat weight. If too much fat is present, the person is considered obese. Obesity long has been recognized as a risk factor for coronary heart disease. Maintaining recommended body weight (fat percent) is essential in any cardiovascular risk reduction program. Guidelines for a comprehensive weight management program are given in Chapter 6.

Blood Lipids

Blood lipids are *fat-soluble substances* in the body. This term is used mainly in reference to cholesterol and triglycerides. Because these substances cannot float around freely in the water-based medium of the blood, they are packaged and transported in the blood by complex molecules called *lipoproteins*.

If you never have had a blood lipid test, it is highly recommended. The blood test includes total cholesterol, high-density lipoprotein cholesterol (HDL-cholesterol), low-density lipoprotein cholesterol (LDL-cholesterol), and triglycerides. A significant elevation in blood lipids has been linked clearly to heart and blood vessel disease.

A poor blood lipid profile is thought to be the most important predisposing factor in the development of CHD, accounting for almost half of all cases. The general recommendation by the National Cholesterol Education Program (NCEP) is to keep total cholesterol levels below 200 mg/dl (see Table 7.2). Cholesterol levels between 200 and 239 mg/dl are borderline high, and levels of 240 mg/dl and above indicate high risk for disease. Approximately 52%, or 94.6 million American adults, have total cholesterol values of 200 mg/dl or higher and 20% have values at or above 240 mg/dl.[7]

Many preventive medicine practitioners recommend a lower total cholesterol level, ranging between 160 and 180 mg/dl. For children the level always should be below 170 mg/dl. In the Framingham Heart Study, a 40-year ongoing

TABLE 7.2 ✤ Standards for Blood Lipids

Total Cholesterol	≤ 200 mg/dl	Desirable
	201–239 mg/dl	Borderline high
	≥ 240 mg/dl	High risk
LDL-Cholesterol	≤ 130 mg/dl	Desirable
	131–159 mg/dl	Borderline high
	≥ 160 mg/dl	High risk
HDL-Cholesterol	≥ 45 mg/dl	Desirable
	36–44 mg/dl	Moderate risk
	≤ 35 mg/dl	High risk
Triglycerides	≤ 125 mg/dl	Desirable
	126–499 mg/dl	Borderline high
	≥ 500 mg/dl	High risk

Source: National Cholesterol Education Program

project in the community of Framingham, Massachusetts, not a single individual with a total cholesterol level of 150 mg/dl or lower has had a heart attack.[8]

Perhaps even more significant is the way cholesterol is carried in the bloodstream. Cholesterol defined as a *waxy substance found only in animal fats and oil*, is transported primarily by high-density and low-density lipoproteins. The high-density lipoproteins (HDL) *tend to attract cholesterol, which is carried to the liver to be metabolized and excreted*. HDLs act as scavengers, removing cholesterol from the body and preventing atherosclerosis, *plaque forming in the arteries*. LDL-cholesterol, on the other hand, *tends to release cholesterol, which then may penetrate the lining of the arteries and speed up the process of atherosclerosis*. The NCEP guidelines state that an LDL-cholesterol value below 130 mg/dl is desirable, between 130 and 159 mg/dl is borderline-high, and 160 mg/dl and above is high risk for cardiovascular disease.

The more HDL-cholesterol, the better. HDL-cholesterol is the "good cholesterol" and offers some protection against heart disease. Evidence suggests that low levels of HDL-cholesterol could be the best predictor of CHD and may be more significant than the total cholesterol value. Substantial research supports the evidence that a low level of HDL-cholesterol has the strongest relationship to CHD at all levels of total cholesterol, including levels below 200 mg/dl. The recommended HDL-cholesterol values to minimize the risk for CHD are 45 mg/dl or higher. A level below 35 mg/dl is viewed as a positive or high risk for CHD. An HDL level above 60 mg/dl is viewed as a negative risk factor, one that decreases the risk of coronary disease.

Increasing the HDL-cholesterol improves the cholesterol profile and decreases the risk for CHD. Habitual aerobic exercise, (intensity level above 6 METs), excessive weight loss, and quitting smoking have all been shown to raise HDL-cholesterol. Getting enough beta-carotene, substituting monounsaturated oils for saturated fat in the diet (not to exceed 30% of all calories consumed during the day), and engaging in drug therapy also promote higher HDL-cholesterol levels.

If LDL-cholesterol is higher than ideal, it can be lowered by losing body fat, taking medication, and manipulating the diet. A diet low in fat, saturated fat, and cholesterol and high in fiber is recommended to decrease LDL-cholesterol. The NCEP recommends replacing saturated fat with monounsaturated fat (for example, olive, canola, peanut, and sesame oils), because the latter does not cause a reduction in HDL-cholesterol and actually may lower LDL-cholesterol.

Many experts believe that, to have a significant effect in lowering LDL-cholesterol, total fat consumption must be significantly lower than the current 30% of total daily caloric intake guideline. When trying to lower LDL-cholesterol, saturated fat consumption should be much lower than the 10% of total daily caloric intake guideline for "healthy" people. Average cholesterol consumption should be well below 300 mg per day.

Saturated fats are found mostly in meats and dairy products but seldom in foods of plant origin. Poultry and fish contain less saturated fat than beef but should be eaten in moderation (about 3 to 6 ounces per day). Unsaturated fats are mainly of plant origin and cannot be converted to cholesterol.

The antioxidant effect of Vitamins C and E and beta-carotene also can reduce the risk for CHD.[9] New information suggests that a single unstable free radical (oxygen compounds produced in normal metabolism) can damage LDL particles. Vitamin C seems to inactivate free radicals, and vitamin E protects LDL from oxidation. Beta-carotene not only absorbs free radicals, keeping them from causing damage, but it also seems to increase HDL levels.

Research studies on the effects of a 30%-fat diet have shown that it has little or no effect in lowering cholesterol and that CHD actually continues to progress in people who have the disease. The good news comes from a 1991 study published in the *Archives of Internal Medicine*,[10] which reported that the men and women in the study lowered their cholesterol by an average of 23% in only 3 weeks following a 10% or less fat-calorie diet combined with a regular aerobic exercise program, primarily walking. In this diet, cholesterol intake was limited to less than 25 mg/day. The author of the study concluded that the exact percent fat guideline (10% or 15%) is unknown (it also varies from individual to individual), but that 30% total fat calories is definitely too high a level when attempting to decrease cholesterol.

A daily 10% total-fat diet requires that the person limit fat intake to an absolute minimum. Some health-care professionals contend that a diet like this is difficult to follow indefinitely. People with high cholesterol levels, however, may not need to follow that diet indefinitely but should adopt the 10% fat diet while attempting to lower cholesterol. Thereafter, eating a 30%-fat-diet may be adequate to maintain recommended cholesterol levels (1991 national data indicate that current fat consumption in the United States averages 37% of total calories; see Figure 5.2 in Chapter 5).

A drawback of very low fat diets (less than 25% fat) is that they tend to lower

HDL-cholesterol and increase triglycerides. If HDL-cholesterol is already low, monounsaturated fat should be added to the diet. Olive oil and nuts are sample food items that are high in monounsaturated fat. A specialized nutrition book should be consulted to determine food items that are high in monounsaturated fat.

The following dietary guidelines are recommended to lower LDL-cholesterol levels:

1. Consume fewer than three eggs per week.

2. Eat red meats (3 ounces per serving) fewer than three times per week, and no organ meats (such as liver and kidneys).

3. Do not eat commercially baked foods.

4. Drink low-fat milk (1% or less fat, preferably) and low-fat dairy products.

5. Do not use coconut oil, palm oil, or cocoa butter.

6. Eat fish instead of red meat.

7. Bake, broil, grill, poach, or steam food instead of frying.

8. Refrigerate cooked meat before adding to other dishes. Remove fat hardened in the refrigerator before mixing the meat with other foods.

9. Avoid fatty sauces made with butter, cream, or cheese.

10. Maintain recommended body weight.

Triglycerides, also known as free fatty acids, in combination with cholesterol, speed up the formation of plaque. Very low-density lipoproteins (VLDLs) and chylomicrons, *carry triglycerides in the blood stream.* These fatty acids are found in poultry skin, lunch meats, and shellfish, but they are manufactured mainly in the liver, from refined sugars, starches, and alcohol. High intake of alcohol and sugars (honey included) significantly raises triglyceride levels. The level can be lowered by cutting down on these foods along with reducing weight (if overweight) and doing aerobic exercise. A normal blood triglyceride level is less than 125 mg/dl (see Table 7.2).

Diabetes

Diabetes mellitus is a *condition in which blood glucose is unable to enter the cells because the pancreas either totally stops producing insulin or does not produce enough to meet the body's needs.* The incidence of cardiovascular disease and death in the diabetic population is quite high. People with chronically elevated blood glucose levels also may have problems in metabolizing fats, which can make them more susceptible to atherosclerosis, increase the risk for coronary disease, and lead to other conditions such as vision loss and kidney damage.

Although diabetes has a genetic predisposition, adult-onset (Type II) diabetes is related closely to overeating, obesity, and lack of physical activity. Approximately 70% of Type II diabetics are overweight or have a history of obesity. In most cases this condition can be corrected through a special diet, a weight-loss program, and a regular exercise program. A diet high in water-soluble fibers (found in fruits, vegetables, oats, and beans) is helpful in treating diabetes. A simple aerobic exercise program (walking, cycling, or swimming four to five times per week) often is prescribed because it increases the body's sensitivity to insulin. Individuals who have high blood glucose levels should consult a physician to decide on the best treatment.

Abnormal Electrocardiograms

The electrocardiogram (ECG or EKG) *provides a record of the electrical impulses that stimulate the heart to contract.* ECGs are taken at rest, during the stress of exercise, and during recovery. An exercise ECG also is known as a graded exercise stress test or a *maximal exercise tolerance test.* Similar to a high-speed road test on a car, a stress ECG reveals the heart's tolerance to high-intensity exercise. Based on the findings, ECGs may be interpreted as normal, equivocal, or abnormal.

A stress ECG frequently is used to diagnose coronary heart disease. It also is administered to determine cardiorespiratory fitness levels, to screen individuals for preventive and cardiac rehabilitation programs, to detect abnormal blood pressure response during exercise, and to establish actual or functional maximal heart rate for exercise prescription purposes.

Not every adult who wishes to start or continue in an exercise program needs a stress ECG. The following guidelines can help you determine when this type of test should be conducted:

1. Men over age 40 and women over age 50.

2. A total cholesterol level above 200 mg/dl, or an HDL-cholesterol level below 35 mg/dl.

3. Hypertensive and diabetic patients.

4. Cigarette smokers.

5. Individuals with a family history of CHD, syncope, or sudden death before age 60.

6. People with an abnormal resting ECG.

7. All individuals with symptoms of chest discomfort, dysrhythmias, syncope, or chronotropic incompetence (a heart rate that increases slowly during exercise and never reaches maximum).

Smoking

More than 47 million adults and 3.5 million adolescents in the United States smoke. Cigarette smoking is the single largest preventable cause of illness and premature death in the United States. When considering all related deaths, tobacco is responsible for 400,000 unnecessary deaths per year. Smoking has been linked to cardiovascular disease, cancer, bronchitis, emphysema, and peptic ulcers.

About 53,000 of those yearly deaths are nonsmokers who were exposed to secondhand smoke in daily life. Both fatal and nonfatal cardiac events are increased greatly in people exposed to passive smoking. Some 37,000 yearly deaths from heart disease are attributed to secondhand smoke. Because of the slight adaptation to the harmful effects of smoking in regular smokers, adverse effects of passive smoking

are much greater to the nonsmoker. Secondhand smoke is ranked behind active smoking and alcohol as the third leading preventable cause of death in the U. S.[11] Passive smoking is a significant risk factor for heart disease in children and adults alike.

In relation to coronary disease, not only does smoking speed up the process of atherosclerosis, but it also produces a threefold increase in the risk of sudden death following a myocardial infarction. Smoking increases heart rate and blood pressure and irritates the heart, which can trigger fatal cardiac arrhythmias (irregular heart rhythms). As far as the extra load on the heart is concerned, giving up one pack of cigarettes per day is the equivalent of losing between 50 and 75 pounds of excess body fat! Another harmful effect is a decrease in HDL-cholesterol, the "good" type that helps control blood lipids.

Pipe and cigar smoking and chewing tobacco also increase the risk for heart disease. Even if no smoke is inhaled, toxic substances are absorbed through the membranes of the mouth and end up in the bloodstream. Individuals who use tobacco in any of these three forms also have a much greater risk for cancer of the oral cavity.

Cigarette smoking, a poor cholesterol profile, low fitness, and high blood pressure are the four major risk factors for coronary disease. The risk for both cardiovascular disease and cancer starts to decrease the moment you quit smoking. The risk approaches that of a lifetime nonsmoker 10 and 15 years, respectively, after cessation.

Quitting cigarette smoking is no easy task. Surveys indicate that nine of 10 smokers want to quit. Only about 20% of smokers who try to quit the first time succeed each year. The addictive properties of nicotine and smoke make quitting difficult. Smokers experience physical and psychological withdrawal symptoms when they stop smoking. Even though giving up smoking can be extremely hard, it is by no means impossible.

The most important factor in quitting cigarette smoking is the person's sincere desire to do so. More than 95% of successful ex-smokers have been able to quit on their own, either by quitting cold turkey or by using self-help kits available from organizations such as the American Cancer Society, the American Heart Association, and the American Lung Association. Only 3% of ex-smokers quit as a result of formal cessation programs. A six-step plan to help people stop smoking is contained in Figure 7.6.

Tension and Stress

Tension and stress have become a normal part of life. Everyone has to deal daily with goals, deadlines, responsibilities, pressures. Almost everything in life (whether positive or negative) can be a source of stress. The stressor itself is not what creates the health hazard but, rather, the individual's response to it. Stress is *the nonspecific response of the human organism to any demand placed upon it.*

The body's response to stress has been the same ever since humans were first put on the earth. Stress prepares the organism to react to the stress-causing event, also called the stressor. Stressors can be biological (illness), psychological (depression, confidence), sociological (winning, losing, peer pressure), and philosophical (spiritual values). The problem, though, is the way in which we react to stress. Many people thrive under stress, whereas others under similar circumstances are unable to handle it. An individual's reaction to a stress-causing agent determines whether stress is positive or negative.

Stress is classified into eustress and distress. In the case of eustress, health and performance continue to improve even as stress increases (positive stress). Distress, on the other hand, refers to the unpleasant or harmful stress under which health and performance begin to deteriorate.

Every person has an optimal level of stress that is most conducive to adequate health and performance. When stress levels reach mental, emotional, and physiological limits, however, eustress becomes distress and the person no longer functions effectively.

Individuals who are under a lot of stress and cannot relax place a constant low-level strain on the cardiovascular system that could manifest itself in the form of heart disease. Further, chronic distress raises the risk for many other health disorders, including hypertension, eating disorders, ulcers, diabetes, asthma, depression, migraine headaches, sleep disorders, and chronic fatigue, and may even play a role in the development of certain types of cancers. Recognizing this turning point and overcoming the problem quickly and efficiently are crucial in maintaining emotional and physiological stability.

Learning to live and get ahead today is virtually impossible without practicing adequate stress management techniques. Perhaps the three most common stress management techniques available are physical exercise, progressive muscle relaxation, and breathing techniques.

Physical Exercise

Physical exercise is one of the simplest tools to control stress. Exercise and fitness are thought to reduce the intensity of the stress response and the recovery time from a stressful event. The value of exercise in reducing stress is related to several factors, the main one being less muscular tension.

For example, a person may be distressed because he or she has a miserable day at work and the job requires 8 hours of work in a smoke-filled room with an intolerable boss. To make matters worse, it is late and on the way home the car in front is going much slower than the speed limit. The body's fight or flight mechanism is activated. *Heart rate and blood pressure shoot up, breathing quickens and deepens, muscles tense up, and all systems say "go."* No action can be initiated, however, or stress dissipated, because you just cannot hit your boss or the car in front of you. A person surely could take action, though, by "hitting" the tennis ball, the weights, the swimming pool, or the jogging trail. By engaging in physical activity, a person is able to reduce the muscular tension and eliminate the physiological changes that triggered the fight-or-flight mechanism.

The following six-step plan has been developed as a guide to help you quit smoking. The total program should be completed in 4 weeks or less. Steps one through four should take no longer than 2 weeks. A maximum of 2 additional weeks are allowed for the rest of the program.

Step One   Decide positively that you want to quit. Now prepare a list of the reasons why you smoke and why you want to quit.

Step Two   Initiate a personal diet and exercise program. Exercise and decreased body weight cause a greater awareness of healthy living and increase motivation for giving up cigarettes.

Step Three   Decide on the approach you will use to stop smoking. You may quit cold turkey or gradually decrease the number of cigarettes smoked daily. Many people have found that quitting cold turkey is the easiest way to do it. Although it may not work the first time, after several attempts, all of a sudden smokers are able to overcome the habit without too much difficulty. Tapering off cigarettes can be done in several ways. You may start by eliminating cigarettes that you do not necessarily need, you can switch to a brand lower in nicotine or tar every couple of days, you can smoke less off each cigarette, or you can simply decrease the total number of cigarettes smoked each day.

Step Four   Set the target date for quitting. In setting the target date, choosing a special date may add a little extra incentive. An upcoming birthday, anniversary, vacation, graduation, family reunion — all are examples of good dates to free yourself from smoking.

Step Five   Stock up on low-calorie foods — carrots, broccoli, cauliflower, celery, popcorn (butter- and salt-free), fruits, sunflower seeds (in the shell), sugarless gum, and plenty of water. Keep such food handy on the day you stop and the first few days following cessation. Replace it for cigarettes when you want one.

Step Six   This is the day that you will quit smoking. On this day and the first few days thereafter, do not keep cigarettes handy. Stay away from friends and events that trigger your desire to smoke. Drink large amounts of water and fruit juices, and eat low-calorie foods. Replace the old behavior with new behavior. You will need to replace smoking time with new positive substitutes that will make smoking difficult or impossible. When you desire a cigarette, take a few deep breaths and then occupy yourself by doing a number of things such as talking to someone else, washing your hands, brushing your teeth, eating a healthy snack, chewing on a straw, doing dishes, playing sports, going for a walk or bike ride, going swimming, and so on.

If you have been successful and stopped smoking, a lot of events still can trigger your urge to smoke. When confronted with such events, people rationalize and think, "One won't hurt." It will not work! Before you know it, you will be back to the regular nasty habit. Be prepared to take action in those situations. Find adequate substitutes for smoking. Remind yourself of how difficult it has been and how long it has taken you to get to this point. As time goes on, it will only get easier rather than worse.

FIGURE 7.6 ❖ Six-step smoking cessation approach.

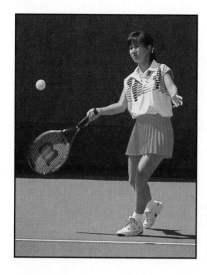

Physical activity is an excellent tool to control stress.

Exercise has enhanced the health and quality of life of millions of people, but for a small group of individuals, exercise can become an obsessive behavior with potentially addictive and overuse properties. Compulsive exercisers often express feelings of guilt and discomfort when they miss a day's workout. Often these individuals continue to exercise even during periods of injury and sickness that require proper rest for adequate recovery. Under these circumstances exercise becomes a biological stressor that will lead to a decrease in health and performance.

As a biological stressor, compulsive exercise or overtraining produces both physiological and psychological symptoms. Almost any type of physical activity (e.g., jogging, basketball, aerobics) performed at very high intensity levels or for unusually prolonged periods (overtraining) can be detrimental to the person's physical and emotional well-being.

Psychological symptoms of overtraining include lower motivation, depression, sleep disturbances, increased irritability, and lack of confidence. Physiological symptoms include musculoskeletal injuries, lower performance, slower recovery time, chronic fatigue, decreased appetite, loss of weight and lean tissue, fat gain, increased muscle tension, higher resting heart rate and blood pressure, and even ECG abnormalities.

If you experience any of these symptoms, you need to reevaluate your exercise program and make adjustments accordingly. People who exceed the recommended guidelines for fitness development and maintenance (see Chapters 3 and 4) are exercising for reasons other than health . . . and some actually may be aggravating an already stressful situation.

Progressive Muscle Relaxation

One of the most popular procedures used to dissipate stress progressive muscle relaxation. This technique enables individuals to relearn the sensation of deep relaxation. It *involves contraction and relaxation of muscle groups throughout the body*. Because chronic stress leads to high muscular tension, being closely aware of how it feels to tighten and relax the muscles progressively will release the tension on the muscles and teach the body to relax at will. Being aware of the tension felt during the exercises also helps the person to be more alert to signs of distress, as similar feelings are experienced in stressful situations. In everyday life these feelings then can be used as a cue to implement relaxation exercises.

Relaxation exercises should be done in a quiet, warm, well-ventilated room. The recommended exercises and the length of the routine vary from one expert to the next. Most important, the person must pay attention to the sensation felt each time the muscles are tensed and relaxed. The exercises should cover all muscle groups. An example of a sequence of progressive muscle relaxation exercises is given in Figure 7.7. The instructions outlined for these exercises can be read to the person, memorized, or tape-recorded. At least 20 minutes should be set aside to perform the entire sequence. Doing relaxation exercises any faster will defeat their purpose. Ideally, a person should repeat the sequence twice a day.

If time is a factor and an individual is not able to go through the entire sequence, only the exercises specific to the area where muscle tension is felt may be done. Performing just a few exercises is better than doing none at all. Of

Stretch out comfortably on the floor, face up, with a pillow under the knees, and assume a passive attitude, allowing the body to relax as much as possible. Contract each muscle group in sequence, taking care to avoid any strain. Muscle tightening should be limited to about 70% of the total possible tension, to prevent cramping or injury to the muscle itself. Paying attention to the sensation of tensing up and relaxing is crucial to produce the relaxation effects. Each contraction is held about 5 seconds, and then the muscles should be allowed to go totally limp. Sufficient time should be allowed for contraction and relaxation before the next instruction.

1. Point your feet, curling the toes downward, and study the tension in the arches and the top of the feet. Hold it and continue to note the tension, then relax. Repeat a second time.

2. Flex the feet upward toward the face and note the tension in your feet and calves. Hold it, and relax. Repeat.

3. Push your heels down against the floor as if burying them in the sand. Hold it and note the tension on the back of the thigh; relax. Repeat one more time.

4. Contract the right thigh by straightening the leg, gently raising the leg off the floor. Hold it and study the tension; relax. Repeat with the left leg; hold and relax. Repeat both legs again.

5. Tense the buttocks by raising your hips ever so slightly off the floor. Hold it and note the tension; relax. Repeat.

6. Contract the abdominal muscles. Hold them tight and note the tension; relax. Repeat one more time.

7. Suck in your stomach — try to make it reach your spine. Flatten your lower back to the floor; hold it and feel the tension in the stomach and lower back; relax. Repeat.

8. Take a deep breath and hold it, then exhale. Repeat. Note your breathing becoming slower and more relaxed.

9. Place your arms on the side of your body and clench both fists. Hold it, study the tension, and relax.

10. Flex the elbow by bringing both hands to the shoulders. Hold it tight and study the tension in the biceps; relax. Repeat.

11. Place your arms flat on the floor, palms up, and push the forearm hard against the floor. Note the tension on the triceps; hold it, and relax. Repeat the exercise.

12. Shrug your shoulders, raising them as high as possible. Hold it and note the tension; relax. Repeat.

13. Gently push your head backward; note the tension in the back of the neck. Hold it, relax. Repeat one more time.

14. Gently bring the head against the chest, push forward, hold, and note the tension in the neck. Relax. Repeat a second time.

15. Press your tongue toward the roof of your mouth. Hold it, study the tension; relax. Repeat.

16. Press your teeth together. Hold it and study the tension; relax. Repeat.

17. Close your eyes tightly. Hold them closed and note the tension. Relax, leaving your eyes closed. Repeat.

18. Wrinkle your forehead. Note the tension; hold it, and relax. Repeat one more time.

FIGURE 7.7 ✤ Progressive muscle relaxation sequence.

course, completing the whole sequence gives the best results.

Breathing Exercises

Breathing techniques also can serve as an antidote to stress. These exercises have been done for centuries in the Orient and India to improve mental, physical, and emotional stamina. The exercises involve *"breathing away" the tension and inhaling fresh air to the entire body.* Breathing exercises can be learned in only a few minutes and require considerably less time than other forms of stress management. An example of these exercises is given in Figure 7.8.

Personal and Family History

Individuals who have a family history of, or already have experienced cardiovascular problems, are at higher risk than those who never have had a problem. People with this sort of history should be encouraged strongly to keep the other risk factors as low as possible. Because most risk factors are reversible, this decreases the risk for future problems significantly.

Age and Gender

Age is a risk factor because of the greater incidence of heart disease in older people. The risk is higher in men over age 45 and women over age 55. This tendency may be induced partly by other factors stemming from changes in lifestyle as we get older (less physical activity, poor nutrition, obesity, and so on). Men are at greater risk for cardiovascular disease than women earlier in life. Following menopause, women's risk increases. Based on final mortality statistics

---

A quiet, pleasant, and well-ventilated room should be used to perform breathing exercises. Any of the three exercises listed below may be done whenever tension is felt due to stress.

Deep breathing	Lie with your back flat against the floor, place a pillow under your knees, feet slightly separated, with toes pointing outward (the exercise also may be conducted sitting up in a chair or standing straight up). Place one hand on your abdomen and the other one on your chest. Slowly breathe in and out so that the hand on your abdomen rises when you inhale and falls as you exhale. The hand on the chest should not move much at all. Repeat the exercise about 10 times. Next, scan your body for tension, and compare your present tension with that felt at the beginning of the exercise. Repeat the entire process once or twice more.
Sighing	Using the abdominal breathing technique, breathe in through your nose to a specific count (e.g., 4, 5, 6). Now exhale through pursed lips to double the intake count (e.g., 10, 11, 12). Repeat the exercise 8 to 10 times whenever you feel tense.
Complete natural breathing:	Sit in an upright position or stand straight up. Breathe through your nose and gradually fill up your lungs from the bottom up. Hold your breath for several seconds. Now exhale slowly by allowing complete relaxation of the chest and abdomen. Repeat the exercise 8 to 10 times.

FIGURE 7.8 ❖ Breathing exercises for stress management.

for 1991, more women (479,359) than men (446,702) died from cardiovascular disease.[12]

Young people should not think that heart disease will not affect them. The process begins early in life. It was shown clearly in American soldiers who died during the Korean and Vietnam conflicts. Autopsies conducted on soldiers killed at 22 years of age and younger revealed that approximately 70% had early stages of atherosclerosis. Other studies found elevated blood cholesterol levels in children as young as 10 years old.

Even though the aging process cannot be stopped, it certainly can be slowed down. Chronological age *(numerical age)* versus functional age *(physiological age)* is an important concept in preventing disease. Some individuals in their 60s or older have the body of a 20-year-old. And 20-year-olds often are in such poor condition and health that they almost seem to have the body of a 60-year-old. Risk factor management and positive lifestyle habits are the best ways to slow down the natural aging process.

CANCER

Cell growth is controlled by deoxyribonucleic acid (DNA) and ribonucleic acid (RNA), *genetic material found in the nucleus of each cell*. When nuclei lose their ability to regulate and control cell growth, cell division is disrupted and mutant cells may develop. Some of these cells may grow uncontrollably and abnormally, forming a mass of tissue called a tumor, which can be either benign or malignant. Benign tumors do not invade other tissue; they are *noncancerous*. They can interfere with normal bodily functions, but they rarely cause death. A malignant tumor is a *cancer*.

Cancer is *a group of diseases characterized by uncontrolled growth and spread of abnormal cells into malignant tumors*. More than 100 types of cancer can develop in any tissue or organ of the human body. Over 23% of all deaths in the United States come from cancer. An estimated 1.2 million new cases are reported, and more than half a million people die each year from cancer.

Cancer cells grow for no reason and multiply, destroying normal tissue. If the spread of cells is not controlled, death ensues. A cell may duplicate as many as 100 times. Normally, the DNA molecule is duplicated perfectly during cell division. In a few cases the DNA molecule is not replicated exactly, but repairs are made quickly by specialized enzymes. Occasionally cells with defective DNA keep dividing and ultimately form a small tumor. As more mutations occur, the altered cells continue to divide and can become malignant. A decade or more can pass between carcinogenic exposure or mutations and the time cancer is diagnosed.

A critical turning point in the development of cancer is when a tumor reaches about one million cells. At this stage it is referred to as carcinoma in situ, an *encapsulated malignant tumor that is found at an early stage and has not spread*. If undetected, the tumor may go for months and years without any significant growth.

While encapsulated, a tumor does not pose a serious threat to human health. To grow, the tumor requires more oxygen and nutrients. In time, a few of the cancer cells start producing chemicals that enhance angiogenesis or *capillary (blood vessel) formation into the tumor*. Angiogenesis is the precursor of metastasis. Metastasis is the *movement of bacteria or body cells from one part of the body to another*. Through these new vessels, cells now can break away from a malignant tumor and migrate to other parts of the body, where they can cause new cancer masses.

Although the immune system and the blood turbulence destroy most cancer cells, only one abnormal cell lodging elsewhere can start a new cancer. These cells also will grow and multiply uncontrollably, destroying normal tissue.

Once cancer cells metastasize, treatment becomes more difficult. Therapy can kill most cancer cells, but a few cells may become resistant to treatment. These cells then can grow into a new tumor that will not respond to the same treatment.

As with cardiovascular disease, cancer is largely preventable. As much as 80% of all human cancer is related to lifestyle or environmental factors (including diet, tobacco use, excessive use of alcohol, sexual and reproductive history, and exposure to occupational hazards).

Equally important is that more than 8 million Americans with a history of cancer were alive in 1995, nearly 5 million of whom were considered cured. For most patients, "cured" means 5 years without symptoms after treatments stop. Life expectancy for these individuals is the same as for those who never have had cancer.[13]

The most effective way to protect against cancer is by changing negative longstanding habits and behaviors. The following general recommendations have been issued in regard to cancer prevention (also see Figure 7.9).

Dietary Changes

The diet should be low in fat and high in fiber and contain vitamins A and C from natural sources. Protein intake should be within the RDA guidelines. Cruciferous vegetables, *plants that produce cross-shaped leaves*, are encouraged. Alcohol should be consumed in moderation, and obesity should be avoided.

High fat intake has been linked primarily to breast, colon, and prostate cancers. Low intake of fiber seems to increase the risk for colon cancer. Foods high in vitamins A and C may deter larynx, esophagus, and lung cancers. Salt-cured, smoked, and nitrite-cured foods have been associated with cancer of the esophagus and stomach. Vitamin C seems to discourage the formation of nitrosamines (cancer-causing substances formed from eating cured meats).

Carrots, squash, sweet potatoes, and cruciferous vegetables (cauliflower, broccoli, cabbage, Brussels sprouts, and kohlrabi) seem to protect against cancer. These vegetables contain a lot of beta-carotene and vitamin C. Researchers believe the antioxidant effect of these vitamins protects the body from oxygen free radicals.

As discussed in Chapter 5, during normal metabolism most of the oxygen in the human body is converted into stable forms of carbon dioxide and water. A small amount, however, ends up in an unstable form known as oxygen free radicals, which are thought to attack and damage the cell membrane and DNA, leading to the formation of cancers. Antioxidants absorb free radicals before they can cause damage, and they also interrupt the sequence of reactions once damage has begun.[14]

A promising new horizon in cancer prevention is the recent discovery of phytochemicals (also see Chapter 5). These chemical compounds, found in abundance in fruits and vegetables, seem to exert a powerful effect in cancer prevention by blocking the formation of cancerous tumors and disrupting the process at almost every step of the way.[15]

As examples of phytochemicals:

❖ Sulforaphane (found in broccoli) removes carcinogens from cells

❖ PEITC (broccoli) and Capsaicin (hot chili peppers) keep carcinogens from binding to DNA

❖ Genistein (soybeans) prevents small tumors from accessing capillaries to get oxygen and nutrients

❖ Flavenoids (most fruits and vegetables) help keep cancer-causing hormones from locking onto cells

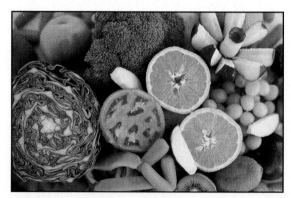

Phytochemicals found in abundance in fruits and vegetables seem to have a powerful effect in decreasing the risk for cancer.

bischlormethyl ether, increase cancer risk. Cigarette smoking magnifies the risk from occupational hazards.

Warning Signals for Cancer

Through early detection, many cancers can be controlled or cured. The real problem is the spreading of cancerous cells. Once that happens, the cancer becomes more difficult to wipe out. Therefore, effective prevention, or at least getting cancer when the possibility of cure is greatest, is crucial. Herein lies the importance of proper periodic screening for prevention and early detection.

Everyone should become familiar with the following seven warning signals for cancer and bring any of them to a physician's attention:

1. Change in bowel or bladder habits.
2. A sore that does not heal.
3. Unusual bleeding or discharge.
4. Thickening or lump in breast or elsewhere.
5. Indigestion or difficulty in swallowing.
6. Obvious change in wart or mole.
7. Nagging cough or hoarseness.

Scientific evidence and testing procedures for prevention and early detection of cancer do change. Studies continue to provide new information about cancer prevention and detection. The intent of cancer prevention programs is to educate and guide individuals toward a lifestyle that will help prevent cancer and enable early detection of malignancy. Treatment of cancer always should be left to specialized physicians and cancer clinics.

CHRONIC OBSTRUCTIVE PULMONARY DISEASE

Chronic obstructive pulmonary disease (COPD) is a term encompassing *diseases that limit air flow*, such as chronic bronchitis, emphysema, and a reactive airway component similar to that of asthma. The incidence of COPD increases proportionately with cigarette smoking (or other forms of tobacco use) and exposure to certain types of industrial pollution. In the case of emphysema, genetic factors also may play a role.

ACCIDENTS

Most people do not consider accidents a health problem, but accidents are the fourth leading cause of death in the United States, affecting the total well-being of millions of Americans each year. Accident prevention and personal safety also are part of a health enhancement program aimed at achieving a higher quality of life. Proper nutrition, exercise, abstinence from cigarette smoking, and stress management are of little help if the person is involved in a disabling or fatal accident caused by distraction, a single reckless decision, or not wearing safety seat belts properly.

Accidents do not just happen. We cause accidents, and we are victims of accidents. Although some factors in life — earthquakes, tornadoes, and airplane crashes for example — are completely beyond our control, more often than not personal safety and accident prevention are a matter of common sense. Most accidents result from poor judgment and confused mental state. Frequently accidents happen when we are upset, not paying attention to the task with which we are involved, or abusing alcohol and other drugs.

Alcohol abuse is the number-one cause of all accidents. Alcohol intoxication is the leading cause of fatal automobile accidents. Other drugs commonly abused in society alter feelings and perceptions, cause mental confusion, and impair judgment and coordination, greatly increasing the risk for accidental morbidity and mortality.

SPIRITUAL WELL-BEING

The National Interfaith Coalition on Aging has defined spiritual well-being, or spirituality as an *affirmation of life in a relationship with God, self, community, and environment that nurtures and celebrates wholeness* (see Figure 7.10). Because this definition encompasses Christians and non-Christians alike, it assumes that all people are spiritual in nature. Spiritual health provides a unifying power that integrates the other dimensions of wellness. Basic characteristics of spiritual people include a sense of meaning and direction in life, a relationship to a higher being, freedom, prayer, faith, love, closeness to others, peace, joy, fulfillment, and altruism (service to others).

Religion has been a major part of cultures since the beginning of time. Although not everyone in the United States claims affiliation with a certain religion or denomination, surveys indicate that over 90% of the U.S. population believes in God or a universal spirit functioning as God.

People, furthermore, believe to a varying extent that (a) a relationship with God is meaningful; (b) God can grant help, guidance, and assistance in daily living; and (c) mortal existence has a purpose. If we accept any or all of these statements, attaining spirituality will have a definite effect on our happiness and well-being.

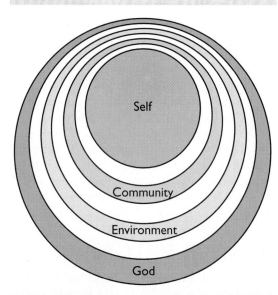

FIGURE 7.10 ❖ Components of spiritual well-being.

Although the reasons why religious affiliation enhances wellness are difficult to determine, possible reasons include the promotion of healthy lifestyle behaviors, social support, assistance in times of crisis and need, and counseling to overcome one's weaknesses.

Altruism, a key attribute of spiritual people, seems to enhance health and longevity. Altruism is defined as *true concern for and action on behalf of others* (opposite of egoism) or a sincere desire to serve others above one's personal needs. Altruism has been the focus of several studies in recent years. Researchers believe that doing good for others is good for oneself, especially for the immune system.

In a study of more than 2,700 people in Michigan,[16] the investigators found that people who did regular volunteer work lived longer. People who did not perform regular volunteer work (at least once a week) had a 250% greater mortality risk during the course of the study. In this same study the authors found that the health benefits of altruism could be so powerful that even just watching films of altruistic endeavors enhances the formation of an immune system chemical that helps fight disease.

Wellness requires a balance between physical, mental, spiritual, emotional, and social well-being. The relationship between spirituality and wellness, therefore, is meaningful in our quest for a better quality of life. As with other parameters of wellness, optimum spirituality requires development of the spiritual nature to its fullest potential.

SUBSTANCE ABUSE CONTROL

Chemical dependencies presently encompasses some of the most serious, self-destructive forms of addiction in our society. Abused substances include alcohol, hard drugs, and cigarettes (the latter already has been discussed in this chapter). Problems associated with substance abuse are drunken or impaired driving, mixing drug prescriptions, family difficulties, and drugs to improve athletic performance (anabolic steroids).

Recognizing that all forms of substance abuse are unhealthy, the following information focuses on three of the most self-destructive addictive substances in our society: alcohol, marijuana, and cocaine.

Alcohol

Alcohol represents one of the most significant health-related drug problems in the United States today. Estimates indicate that seven in 10 adults, or more than 100 million Americans 18 years and older, are drinkers. Approximately 10 million of them will have a drinking problem, including alcoholism, in their lifetime. Another 3 million teenagers are thought to have a drinking problem.

Alcohol intake cuts down peripheral vision, impairs the ability to see and hear, causes slower reactions, reduces concentration and motor performance (including swaying and poor judgment of distance and speed of moving objects), lessens fear, increases risk-taking behaviors, causes more frequent urination, and induces sleep. A single large dose of alcohol may lower sexual function. One of the most unpleasant, dangerous, and life-threatening consequences of drinking is the synergistic action of alcohol when combined with other drugs, particularly central nervous system depressants.

Long-term manifestations of alcohol abuse can be serious and life-threatening. These conditions include cirrhosis of the liver (scarring of the liver, often fatal); greater risk for oral, esophageal, and liver cancer; cardiomyopathy (a disease that affects the heart muscle); high blood pressure; greater risk for strokes; inflammation of the esophagus, stomach, small intestine, and pancreas; stomach ulcers; sexual impotence; malnutrition; brain cell damage and consequent loss of memory; psychosis; depression; and hallucinations.

Hard Drugs

Approximately 60% of the world's production of illegal drugs is consumed in the United States.

Each year Americans spend more than $100 billion on illegal drugs, surpassing the total dollars taken in from all crops produced by U.S. farmers. According to the U.S. Department of Education, today's drugs are stronger and more addictive, posing a greater risk than ever before. Drugs lead to physical and psychological dependence. If used regularly, they integrate into the body's chemistry, raising drug tolerance and forcing the person to increase the dosage constantly for similar results. In addition to the serious health problems caused by drug abuse, more than half of all adolescent suicides are drug-related.

Marijuana

Marijuana (pot or grass) is the most widely used illegal drug in the United States. Approximately 20 million people in the country use marijuana regularly. Earlier studies in the 1960s indicated that the potential effects of marijuana were exaggerated and that the drug was relatively harmless. The drug as it is used today, however, is as much as 10 times stronger than it was when the initial studies were conducted. Long-term harmful effects of marijuana use include atrophy of the brain, leading to irreversible brain damage, decreased resistance to infectious diseases, chronic bronchitis, lung cancer, and possible sterility and impotence.

Cocaine

Similar to marijuana, for many years cocaine was thought to be a relatively harmless drug. This misconception came to an abrupt halt in 1986 when two well-known athletes, Len Bias (basketball) and Don Rogers (football), died suddenly following a cocaine overdose. An estimated 4 to 6 million Americans use cocaine, 96% of whom had used marijuana previously.

Sustained cocaine snorting can lead to a constant runny nose, nasal congestion and inflammation, and perforation of the nasal septum. Long-term consequences of cocaine use in general include loss of appetite, digestive disorders, weight loss, malnutrition, insomnia, confusion, anxiety, and cocaine psychosis (characterized by paranoia and hallucinations). Large overdoses of cocaine end in sudden death from respiratory paralysis, cardiac arrhythmias, and severe convulsions. Some individuals lack an enzyme used in metabolizing cocaine, and for them as few as two to three lines of cocaine may be fatal.

Recognizing the hazards of chemical use, families, teams, and communities can assist each other in preventing problems, as well as help those who have problems with chemical use. Moreover, treating chemical dependency (including alcohol) seldom is accomplished without professional guidance and support. To secure the best available assistance, people in need should contact a physician or obtain a referral from a local mental health clinic (see Yellow Pages in the phone book.)

SEXUALLY TRANSMITTED DISEASES

As the name implies, sexually transmitted diseases (STDs) are *diseases spread through sexual contact*. STDs have reached epidemic proportions in the United States. Of the more than 25 known STDs, some are still incurable. The American Social Health Association stated that 25% of all Americans will acquire at least one STD in their lifetime. Each year more than 12 million people are newly infected with STDs, including 4.6 million cases of chlamydia, 1.8 million of gonorrhea, 1 million of genital warts, half a million of herpes, and nearly 100,000 cases of syphilis. Attracting most of the attention because of its life-threatening potential were more than 80,691 new cases of AIDS in the United States in 1994.

AIDS is the most frightening of all STDs because it has no known cure and none is predicted for the near future. AIDS, which stands for acquired immunodeficiency syndrome, is the *end stage of infection by the human immunodeficiency virus.*

The human immunodeficiency virus (HIV) is a *chronic infectious disease that spreads among individuals who engage in risky behavior such as unprotected sex or the sharing of hypodermic needles*. When a person becomes infected with HIV, the virus multiplies and attacks and destroys white blood cells. These cells are part of the immune system, and their function is to fight off infections and diseases in the body.

As the number of white blood cells killed increases, the body's immune system breaks down gradually or may be destroyed totally. Without the immune system a person becomes susceptible to opportunistic infections or cancers not ordinarily seen in healthy people.

HIV is a progressive disease. At first, people who become infected with HIV may not know they are infected. An incubation period of weeks, months, or years may go by during which time no symptoms appear. The virus may live in the body 10 years or longer before symptoms emerge. As of 1994, almost 44% of the people infected with HIV in the United States did not know they were infected until they began developing AIDS-related symptoms.[17]

As the infection progresses to the point at which certain diseases develop, the person is said to have AIDS. HIV itself doesn't kill. Nor do people die from AIDS. AIDS is the term used to define the final stage of HIV infection. Death is caused by a weakened immune system that is unable to fight off opportunistic diseases.

On the average, 7 to 8 years elapse after infection before the individual develops the symptoms that fit the case definition of AIDS. From that point on, the person may live another 2 to 3 years. In essence, from the point of infection, the individual may endure a chronic disease for 8 to 10 years.

No one has to become infected with HIV. Once infected with the virus, a person will never become uninfected. There is no second chance. Everyone must protect himself or herself against this chronic disease. No one should be so ignorant as to believe that it can never happen to him or her!

HIV is transmitted by the exchange of cellular body fluids — blood, semen, vaginal secretions, and maternal milk. These fluids may be exchanged during sexual intercourse, by using hypodermic needles used previously by infected individuals, between a pregnant woman and her developing fetus, babies from an infected mother during childbirth, less frequently during breast feeding, and rarely from a blood transfusion or organ transplant.

AIDS is an "equal opportunity epidemic." People do not get HIV because of who they are but, rather, because of what they do. HIV and AIDS threaten anyone, anywhere: men, women, children, teenagers, young people, older adults, Whites, Blacks, Hispanics, Asians, homosexuals, heterosexuals, bisexuals, druggies, Americans, Africans, Europeans. Nobody is immune to HIV.

You cannot tell if people are infected with HIV or have AIDS simply by looking at them or taking their word. Not you, not a nurse, not even a doctor can tell, unless an HIV antibody test is done. Therefore, every time you engage in risky behavior, you run the risk of contracting HIV. The two most basic risky behaviors are: (a) having unprotected vaginal, anal, or oral sex with an HIV-infected person, and (b) sharing hypodermic needles or other drug paraphernalia with someone who is infected.

The Centers for Disease Control and Prevention estimate that 1 million Americans are infected with HIV. Because of the lengthy incubation period (7 to 8 years to develop AIDS), about 20% of the AIDS patients today are believed to have been infected as teenagers. By the end of 1993, a total of 357,916 AIDS cases had been diagnosed in the United States and 171,980 had died from the diseases caused by HIV. The number of deaths is expected to double in 3 years. Most of the people who die are in the 20- to 45-year-old age group. By the year 2000, HIV infection will become the third leading cause of death in the United States, behind cardiovascular diseases and cancer.

Approximately 66% of all AIDS cases in the United States have occurred in gay or bisexual men. AIDS in heterosexuals, nonetheless, is on the rise and now is spreading at a faster rate in heterosexuals. Many heterosexuals practice unprotected sex because they don't believe it can happen to their segment of the population. HIV is an epidemic that does not discriminate by sexual orientation. Worldwide about 75% of the AIDS cases have been reported in heterosexuals.

As with any other serious illness, AIDS patients deserve respect, understanding, and support. Rejection and discrimination are traits of immature, hateful, and ignorant people. Education, knowledge, and responsible behaviors are the best ways to minimize fear and discrimination.

The best way to prevent sexually transmitted diseases is through a mutually monogamous sexual relationship, sex with only one person who has sexual relations only with you. Risky behaviors that significantly increase the chances of contracting sexually transmitted diseases, including HIV infection, are:

1. Multiple or anonymous sexual partners such as a pickup or prostitute.
2. Anal sex with or without a condom.
3. Vaginal or oral sex with someone who shoots drugs or engages in anal sex.
4. Sex with someone you know who has several sex partners.
5. Unprotected sex (without a condom) with an infected person.
6. Sexual contact of any kind with anyone who has symptoms of AIDS or who is a member of a high-risk group for AIDS.

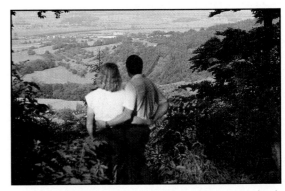

A monogamous sexual relationship almost completely removes people from risking HIV infection and the danger of developing other sexually transmitted diseases.

7. Sharing toothbrushes, razors, or other implements that could become contaminated with blood with anyone who is, or might be, infected with the HIV virus.

Avoiding risky behaviors that destroy quality of life and life itself are critical components of a healthy lifestyle. Learning the facts so you can make responsible choices can protect you and those around you from startling and unexpected conditions. Using alcohol moderately (or not at all), refraining from substance abuse, and preventing sexually transmitted diseases are keys to averting both physical and psychological damage.

NOTES

1. U. S. Department of Health and Human Services, National Center for Health Statistics, *Monthly Vital Statistics Report: Advance Report of Final Mortality Statistics*, 43:6, Supplement (1992), March 22, 1995.
2. J. M. McGinnis and W. H. Foege, "Actual Causes of Death in the United States." *Journal of the American Medical Association* 270 (1993), 2207–2212.
3. American Heart Association, *Heart and Stroke Facts: 1995* (Statistical Supplement) (Dallas: AHA, 1994).
4. U. S. Department of Health and Human Services.
5. P. N. Hopkins and R. R. Williams, "Identification and Relative Weight of Cardiovascular Risk Factors," *Cardiology Clinics*, 4 (1986), 3–32.

6. S. N. Blair, H. W. Kohl III, R. S. Paffenbarger, Jr., D. G. Clark, K. H. Cooper, and L. W. Gibbons, "Physical Fitness and All-Cause Mortality: A Prospective Study of Healthy Men and Women," *Journal of the American Medical Association*, 262 (1989), 2395–2401.
7. American Heart Association, *Fact Sheet on Heart Attack, Stroke and Risk Factors* (Dallas: AHA, 1994).
8. W. P. Castelli and K. Anderson, "A Population at Risk. Prevalence of High Cholesterol Levels in Hypertensive Patients in the Framingham Study," *American Journal of Medicine* 80, Supplement 2A (1986), 23-32.
9. J. M. Gaziano and C. H. Hennekens, "A New Look at What Can Unclog Your Arteries," *Executive Health Report*, 27:8 (1991), 16.

10. R. J. Barnard, "Effects of Lifestyle Modification on Serum Lipids," *Archives of Internal Medicine*, 151 (1991), 1389–1394.
11. S. A. Glantz and W. W. Parmley. "Passive Smoking and Heart Disease," *Journal of the American Medical Association*, 273 (1995), 1047–1053.
12. American Heart Association.
13. American Cancer Society. *1995 Cancer Facts and Figures* (New York: ACS, 1995).
14. Gaziano and Hennekens.
15. S. Begley. "Beyond Vitamins." *Newsweek*, April 25, 1994, pp. 45–49.
16. E. R. Growald and A. Lusks, "Beyond Self." *American Health*, March 1988, pp. 51-53.
17. E. Pennisi, "AIDS Becomes More of an Equal Opportunity Epidemic," *American Society for Microbiology News* 61:5 (1995), 236-240.

Relevant Questions and Answers to Fitness and Wellness

CHAPTER 8

KEY TERMS

Amenorrhea

Anabolic steroids

Calorie

Concentric muscle
contraction

Eccentric muscle
contraction

Exercise intolerance

Heat cramps

Heat exhaustion

Heat stroke

Kilocalorie

Muscle hypertrophy

Oligomenorrhea

Osteoporosis

Shin splint

Side stitch

OBJECTIVES

❖ Dispel some misconceptions related to physical fitness
and wellness.

❖ To give practical advice and tips regarding safety.

❖ To address some concerns specific to women.

❖ To clarify some concepts regarding nutrition and
weight control.

❖ To provide guidelines related to fitness/wellness
consumer issues.

*S*ome of the most frequently asked questions regarding various aspects of physical fitness and wellness are addressed in this chapter. The answers
will further clarify concepts discussed throughout the
book, as well as put to rest several myths that misin-
form fitness and wellness participants.

SAFETY OF EXERCISE PARTICIPATION AND INJURY PREVENTION

Q *Can aerobic exercise make a person immune to heart and
blood vessel disease?*

A Scientific evidence clearly indicates that aerobically fit individuals have a much lower incidence of cardiovascular

disease. A regular aerobic exercise program by itself, however, is not an absolute guarantee against diseases of the heart and blood vessels. Several factors increase a person's risk for cardiovascular disease.

Though physical inactivity is one of the most significant risk factors, studies have documented that multiple interrelations usually exist between these risk factors. Physical inactivity, for instance, often contributes to an increase in (a) body fat, (b) LDL-cholesterol, (c) triglycerides, (d) tension and stress, (e) blood pressure, and (f) risk for diabetes (see Figure 8.1). As discussed in Chapter 7, most risk factors are preventable and reversible. Overall risk factor management is the best advice to minimize the risk for cardiovascular disease. Research also indicates that the odds of surviving a heart attack are much higher for people who engage in a regular aerobic exercise program.

Q *What amount of aerobic exercise is optimal for decreasing the risk for cardiovascular disease significantly?*

A The required amount of exercise to maintain cardiorespiratory fitness is a training session approximately every 48 hours for 20 to 30 minutes in the appropriate target training zone. Although aerobic exercise definitely reduces the risk for cardiovascular problems, the amount of exercise required to offset the risk cannot be pinpointed specifically because of the many individual differences (genetic and lifestyle) between people.

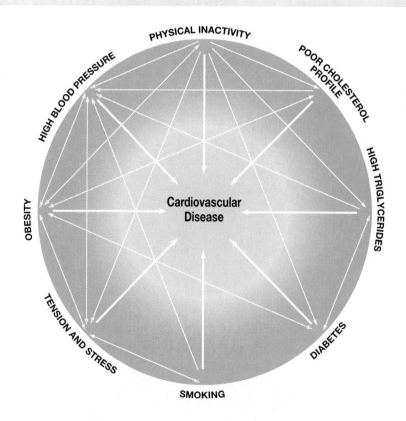

FIGURE 8.1 ❖ Interrelationships among leading cardiovascular risk factors.

Fitness & Wellness

According to some data,[1] about 300 calories should be expended daily through aerobic exercise to obtain a certain degree of protection against cardiovascular disease. Dr. Ralph Paffenbarger and his co-researchers' study on Harvard alumni (see Figure 1.5 in Chapter 1) found that expending 2,000 calories per week as a result of physical activity yielded the lowest risk for cardiovascular disease in this group of almost 17,000 alumni (2,000 calories per week represents about 300 calories per daily exercise session).

The work alluded to in Chapter 7 (see Figure 7.6) conducted at the Aerobics Research Institute in Dallas indicated that even moderate fitness levels can reduce the incidence of cardiovascular problems substantially. The minimum dose for moderate fitness requires an expenditure of about 200 calories five to seven times per week. Slightly greater protection is achieved at higher fitness levels. As noted in the previous question, exercise by itself does not provide an absolutely risk-free guarantee against cardiovascular disease.

Q *At what age should I start concerning myself with cardiovascular disease?*

A The disease process, not only for cardiovascular disease but also cancer, starts early in life as a result of poor lifestyle habits. Studies

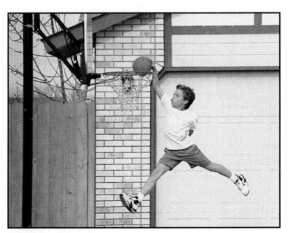

Regular physical activity during youth enhances the likelihood of lifetime participation in an exercise program.

have shown beginning stages of atherosclerosis and elevated blood lipids in children as young as 10 years old.

Many positive habits can be established early in life within the walls of one's own home. If people are taught at a young age that they should avoid excessive calories, sweets, salt, alcohol; not to use tobacco; and participate in physical activity; their chances of leading a healthier life are much greater than is true with the present generation. Some of the best advice to humanity when it comes to teaching is: "Come and follow me." If you cultivate positive health habits in your own life, your children will be more likely to follow.

Q *Can I exercise after donating blood?*

A The average amount of blood taken in donations is about 500 ml (half liter) of a total body volume of 5 liters. This volume is replenished immediately by reserve blood components stored in the body. Unless you are given special instructions not to exercise, there is no reason you cannot continue with your regular program.

Q *Will exercise offset the detrimental effects of cigarette smoking?*

A Physical exercise often motivates toward smoking cessation but does not offset any ill effects of smoking. Smoking greatly decreases the ability of the blood to transport oxygen to working muscles. *Oxygen is carried in the circulatory system* by hemoglobin, the iron-containing pigment of the red blood cells. Carbon monoxide, a byproduct of cigarette smoke, has 210 to 250 times greater affinity for hemoglobin than oxygen does. Consequently, carbon monoxide combines much faster with hemoglobin, decreasing the oxygen-carrying capacity of the blood.

Chronic smoking also increases airway resistance, requiring the respiratory muscles to work much harder and consume more oxygen to ventilate a given amount of air. If you quit smoking, exercise does help increase the functional capacity of the pulmonary system.

Q Will exercise help me feel better?

A Yes, many studies have found that exercise helps people feel better, improve self-esteem and self-confidence, relieve stress, and even reduce depression. As with the physiological benefits of exercise, psychological benefits are enjoyed through regular participation. Hence, a lifetime of physical activity is just as important for mental wellness.

Q How can I tell if I'm exceeding the safe limits for exercising?

A The best method to determine whether you are exercising too strenuously is to check your heart rate and make sure it does not exceed the limits of your target zone. Exercising above this target zone may not be safe for unconditioned or high-risk individuals. You do not need to exercise beyond your target zone to gain the desired benefits for the cardiorespiratory system.

In addition, several physical signs will tell you when you are exceeding functional limitations: rapid or irregular heart rate, difficult breathing, nausea, vomiting, lightheadedness, headaches, dizziness, pale skin, flushness, extreme weakness, lack of energy, shakiness, sore muscles, cramps, and tightness in the chest. These are all signs of exercise intolerance, the *physical aversion to exercise conducted at intensity levels beyond a person's functional capacity.* Learn to listen to your body. If you notice any of these symptoms, seek medical attention before continuing your exercise program.

Q How fast should heart rate decrease following aerobic exercise?

A To a certain extent, recovery heart rate is related to fitness level. The better your cardiorespiratory fitness level, the faster your heart rate will decrease following exercise. As a rule of thumb, heart rate should be below 120 beats per minute 5 minutes into recovery. If your heart rate is above 120, you most likely have overexerted yourself or possibly could have some other cardiac abnormality. If you decrease the intensity or duration of exercise, or both, and you still have a fast heart rate 5 minutes into recovery, consult your physician.

Q How fast does a person lose the benefits of exercise after stopping an exercise program?

A How quickly the benefits of exercise are lost differs among the various components of physical fitness and also depends on the condition the person achieves before discontinuing the exercise. Specifically with regard to cardiorespiratory endurance, it has been estimated that 4 weeks of aerobic training are completely reversed in 2 consecutive weeks of physical inactivity.

On the other hand, if you have been exercising regularly for months or years, 2 weeks of inactivity will not hurt you as much as it will someone who has exercised only a few weeks. Generally speaking, within 48 to 72 hours of aerobic inactivity, the cardiorespiratory system starts to lose some of its capacity. Flexibility can be maintained with two or three stretching sessions per week, and strength is easily maintained with just one maximal training session per week. If you have to interrupt the program for reasons beyond your control, do not attempt to resume your training at the same level you left off but, instead, build up gradually again.

A regular fitness program should be maintained even during traveling and vacation periods. When traveling, plan ahead and examine your options before you leave home. Many hotels provide in-house fitness facilities. Although the equipment often is limited, it's generally sufficient for an adequate cardiorespiratory and strength workout. Frequent travelers would benefit from joining a nationally franchised health club, a YMCA, or a YWCA. In this manner you can continue the same exercise program while visiting different cities.

Activities that require a minimum of equipment and no facilities, such as jogging or rope jumping, are excellent alternatives for the road. If you are going to venture out in a new city, always ask for safe places to jog. Nearby parks or a high school track are usually safe and help you stay away from traffic and stoplights. The strength-training (without equipment) and flexibility exercises provided in Appendices B and C can be used to maintain your strength and flexibility. If visiting a resort area, fitness rental equipment, such as bikes or roller blades is often available.

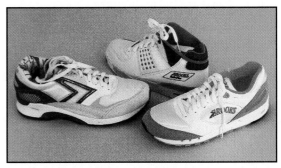

Activity-specific shoes are recommended to prevent lower extremity injuries.

Q *What type of clothing should I wear when I exercise?*

A The type of clothing you wear during exercise is important. In general, clothing should fit comfortably and allow free movement of the various body parts. Select clothing according to air temperature, humidity, and exercise intensity. Avoid nylon and rubberized materials and tight clothes that interfere with the cooling mechanism of the human body or obstruct normal blood flow. Fabrics made from polypropylene, Capilene, Thermax, and synthetics are best. These types of fabrics draw moisture away from the skin, enhancing evaporation and cooling of the body. Exercise intensity is also important because the harder you exercise, the more heat the body produces.

When exercising in the heat, avoid the hottest time of the day, between 11:00 a.m. and 5:00 p.m. Surfaces such as asphalt, concrete, and artificial turfs should be avoided because they absorb heat, which then radiates to the body. (Also see the discussion on exercise in hot and humid conditions in this chapter).

Only a minimal amount of clothing is necessary during exercise in the heat, to allow for maximal evaporation. Clothing should be lightweight, light-colored, loose-fitting, airy, and absorbent. Examples of commercially available products that can be used during exercise in the heat include Asci's Perma Plus, Cool-max, and Nike's Dri-F.I.T. Double-layer acrylic socks are more absorbent than cotton and help to prevent blistering and chafing of the feet. A straw-type hat can be worn to protect the eyes and head from the sun. Clothing for exercise in the cold is discussed later in this chapter.

A good pair of shoes is vital to prevent lower-limb injuries. Shoes manufactured specifically for your choice of activity are a must. Body type, tendency toward pronation or supination, and exercise surfaces must be considered when selecting proper footwear. Shoes should have good stability, motion control, and comfortable fit. Purchase shoes in the middle of the day when feet have expanded and might be one-half size larger. For increased breathability, choose shoes with nylon or mesh uppers. Generally, salespeople at reputable athletic shoe stores are knowledgeable and can help select a good shoe that fits your needs. Examine your shoes after 500 miles or 6 months, and obtain a new pair if they are worn out. Old shoes frequently are responsible for lower-limb injuries.

Q *What time of the day is best for exercise?*

A A person can exercise at almost any time of the day except about 2 hours following a regular meal, or the noon and early afternoon hours on hot and humid days. Many people enjoy exercising early in the morning because it gives them a good boost to start the day. Others prefer the lunch hour for weight-control reasons. By exercising at noon, they do not eat as big a lunch, which helps keep down daily caloric intake. Highly stressed people seem to like the evening hours because of the relaxing effects of exercise.

Q How long should a person wait after a meal before engaging in strenuous physical exercise?

A The length of time to wait before exercising after a meal depends on the amount of food eaten. On the average, after a regular meal a person should wait about 2 hours before participating in strenuous physical activity. Light physical activity, such as a walk, is fine. If anything, it helps burn extra calories and may help the body metabolize fats more efficiently.

Q How should acute sports injuries be treated?

A The best treatment always has been prevention itself. If an activity is causing unusual discomfort or chronic irritation, attend to the cause by decreasing the intensity, switching activities, or using better equipment such as properly-fitting shoes.

In the case of an acute injury, the standard method of treatment is (a) cold application, (b) compression or splinting, or both, and (c) elevation of the affected body part. Cold should be applied three to five times a day for 15 to 20 minutes at a time during the first 24 to 36 hours. This can be done by submerging the injured area in cold water and gradually adding ice to it or using an icebag or applying ice massage to the affected part. Compression can be applied with an elastic bandage or wrap (not too tight). Elevating the body part, whenever possible, decreases blood flow to it. The purpose of these three types of treatment is to minimize swelling in the area, which greatly increases recovery time.

After the first 36 to 48 hours, heat can be applied if no further swelling or inflammation occurs. If you have doubts regarding the nature or seriousness of the injury (such as suspected fracture), you should seek a medical evaluation.

Whenever a deformity (such as in fractures, dislocations, or partial dislocations) is obvious, splinting, cold application with an icebag, and medical attention are required. Never try to reset any of these conditions by yourself, as you could further damage muscles, ligaments, and nerves. Treatment of these injuries always should be left to specialized medical personnel. A quick reference guide for the signs or symptoms and treatment of exercise-related problems is provided in Table 8.1.

Q What causes muscle soreness and stiffness?

A Muscle soreness and stiffness are common in individuals who (a) begin an exercise program or participate after a long layoff from exercise, (b) exercise beyond their customary intensity and duration, and (c) perform eccentric training. The acute soreness that sets in the first few hours after exercise is thought to be related to a lack of blood (oxygen) flow and general fatigue of the exercised muscles. The delayed soreness that appears several hours after exercise (usually 12 hours or so later) and lasts 2 to 4 days may be related to actual tiny tears in muscle tissue, muscle spasms that increase fluid retention stimulating the pain nerve endings, and overstretching or tearing of connective tissue in and around muscles and joints.

Two types of contraction accompany muscular activity with movement (isotonic contractions, see Chapter 3): concentric and eccentric. During a concentric muscle contraction the *muscle shortens as it develops tension*. In eccentric muscle contraction the *muscle fibers lengthen while developing tension*.

For example, during the arm-curl exercise the elbow flexor muscles (biceps, brachioradialis, and brachialis) shorten as the weight is brought toward the shoulder (concentric contractions). On the way down the muscles contract eccentrically as they lengthen while the person lowers the weight slowly to the starting position. Similarly, running downhill requires eccentric

TABLE 8.1 ❖ Reference Guide for Exercise-Related Problems

Injury	Signs/Symptoms	Treatment*
Bruise (contusion)	Pain, swelling, discoloration	Cold application, compression, rest
Dislocations/ Fractures	Pain, swelling, deformity	Splinting, cold application, seek medical attention
Heat cramps	Cramps, spasms and muscle twitching in the legs, arms, and abdomen	Stop activity, get out of the heat, stretch, massage the painful area, drink plenty of fluids
Heat exhaustion	Fainting, profuse sweating, cold/clammy skin, weak/rapid pulse, weakness, headache	Stop activity, rest in a cool place, loosen clothing, rub body with cool/wet towel, drink plenty of fluids, stay out of heat for 2–3 days
Heat stroke	Hot/dry skin, no sweating, serious disorientation, rapid/full pulse, vomiting, diarrhea, unconsciousness, high body temperature	*Seek* immediate medical attention, request help and get out of the sun, bathe in cold water/spray with cold water/rub body with cold towels, drink plenty of cold fluids
Joint sprains	Pain, tenderness, swelling, loss of use, discoloration	Cold application, compression, elevation, rest, heat after 36 to 48 hours (if no further swelling)
Muscle cramps	Pain, spasm	Stretch muscle(s), use mild exercises for involved area
Muscle soreness and stiffness	Tenderness, pain	Mild stretching, low-intensity exercise, warm bath
Muscle strains	Pain, tenderness, swelling, loss of use	Cold application, compression, elevation, rest, heat after 36 to 48 hours (if no further swelling)
Shin splints	Pain, tenderness	Cold application prior to and following any physical activity, rest, heat (if no activity is carried out)
Side stitch	Pain on the side of the abdomen below the rib cage	Decrease level of physical activity or stop altogether, gradually increase level of fitness
Tendinitis	Pain, tenderness, loss of use	Rest, cold application, heat after 48 hours

* Cold should be applied 3 to 4 times a day for 15 minutes.
  Heat can be applied 3 times a day for 15 to 20 minutes.

contractions in the leg muscles, and level running requires concentric contractions. Eccentric training has been shown to produce more muscle soreness than concentric training.

To prevent soreness and stiffness, the recommended approach is to warm up gradually before physical activity and stretch adequately after exercise. Do not attempt to do too much too quickly. If you become sore and stiff, mild stretching, low-intensity exercise to stimulate blood flow, and a warm bath can help relieve the pain.

Stretching may be of greatest significance following exercise. Tired muscles tend to contract to a shorter than normal length. Byproducts of exercise metabolism also may cause muscle spasms. Post-exercise stretching thus can help return a muscle to its normal length.

Q How should I care for shin splints?

A One of the most common injuries to the lower limbs is the shin splint. This is a *condition characterized by pain and irritation in the shin region of the leg*. It usually results from one or more of the following: (a) lack of proper and gradual conditioning, (b) doing physical activities on hard surfaces (wooden floors, hard tracks, cement, and asphalt), (c) fallen arches in the feet, (d) chronic overuse, (e) muscle fatigue, (f) faulty posture, (g) improper shoes, and (h) excessively overweight while participating in weight-bearing activities.

Shin splints may be managed by:

— removing or reducing the cause (exercising on softer surfaces, wearing better shoes or arch supports, or completely stopping that exercise modality until the shin splints heal)

— doing mild stretching exercises before and after physical activity

— using ice massage for 10 to 20 minutes before and after physical participation

— applying active heat (whirlpool and hot baths) for 15 minutes, two to three times a day.

In addition, supportive taping during physical activity is helpful (a qualified athletic trainer can readily teach you the proper taping technique).

Q What causes side stitch?

A Side stitch happens primarily in the early stages of exercise participation. The exact cause of this *sharp pain in the side that occurs sometimes during exercise* is unknown. Some experts suggest that it could relate to a lack of blood flow to the respiratory muscles during strenuous physical exertion. Side stitch occurs primarily in unconditioned beginners and in trained individuals when they exercise at higher intensities than usual. As one's physical condition improves, this problem disappears unless training is intensified. Some people, however, encounter side stitch during downhill running. If side stitch is a problem for you, slow down, and if it persists, stop altogether. Lying down on your back and gently bringing both knees to the chest and holding that position for 30 to 60 seconds also helps.

Some people also get side stitch if they eat or drink juice shortly before exercise. Drinking only water an hour to two prior to exercise can prevent side stitch. Other individuals have problems with commercially available carbohydrate solutions during high-intensity exercise. Unless carbohydrate replacement is crucial to complete an event (marathon, triathlon), drink cool water for fluid replacement, or try a different carbohydrate solution. Fluid and carbohydrate replacement during prolonged exercise or exercise in the heat are discussed later in this chapter.

Q What causes muscle cramps, and what should be done when they occur?

A Muscle cramps are caused by the body's depletion of essential electrolytes or a breakdown in coordination between opposing muscle groups. If you have a muscle cramp, first attempt to stretch the muscles involved. In the case of the calf muscle, for example, pull your toes up toward the knees. After stretching the affected muscles, gently rub them down, and finally do some mild exercises requiring the use of those particular muscles.

In pregnant and lactating women muscle cramps often are related to a lack of calcium. If women get cramps during these times, calcium supplements usually relieve the problem. Tight clothing also can cause cramps because it restricts blood flow to active muscle tissue.

Q *Why is exercising in hot and humid conditions unsafe?*

A When a person exercises, only 30%–40% of the energy the body produces is used for mechanical work or movement. The rest of the energy (60%–70%) is converted into heat. If this heat cannot be dissipated properly because the weather is too hot or the relative humidity is too high, body temperature increases and in extreme cases can result in death.

The specific heat of body tissue (the heat required to raise the temperature of the body by 1°C) is .38 calories per pound of body weight per 1°C (.38 cal/lb/°C). This indicates that if no body heat is dissipated, a 150-pound person has to burn only 57 calories (150 × .38) to increase total body temperature by 1°C. If this person were to engage in an exercise session requiring 300 calories (about 3 miles running) without dissipating any heat, the inner body temperature would increase by 5.3°C, the equivalent of going from 98.6 to 108.1°F.

This example clearly illustrates the need for caution when exercising in hot or humid weather. If the relative humidity is too high, body heat cannot be lost through evaporation because the atmosphere already is saturated with water vapor. In one instance, a football casualty occurred at a temperature of only 64°F but at a relative humidity of 100%. As a general rule, care must be taken when air temperature is above 90°F and relative humidity is above 60%.

The American College of Sports Medicine has recommended that individuals should not engage in strenuous physical activity when the readings of a wet bulb globe thermometer exceed 82.4°F. With this type of thermometer, the wet bulb is cooled by evaporation, and on dry days it shows a lower temperature than the regular (dry) thermometer. On humid days the cooling effect is less because of decreased evaporation; hence, the difference between the wet and dry readings is not as great.

The American Running and Fitness Association offers the following descriptions and first-aid measures for the three major signs of trouble when exercising in the heat:

1. **Heat cramps.** *Symptoms include cramps and spasms and muscle twitching in the legs, arms, and abdomen.* To relieve heat cramps, stop exercising, get out of the heat, massage the painful area, slowly stretch, and drink plenty of fluids.

2. **Heat exhaustion.** *Symptoms include fainting, dizziness, profuse sweating, cold, clammy skin, weakness, headache, and a rapid, weak pulse.* If you incur any of these symptoms, stop and find a cool place to rest. Drink plenty of cool fluids. Loosen or remove clothing, and rub your body with a cool, wet towel. Stay out of the heat for the rest of the day and possibly for the next 2 or 3 days.

3. **Heat stroke.** *Symptoms include serious disorientation; warm, dry skin; no sweating; rapid, full pulse; vomiting; diarrhea; unconsciousness; and high body temperature.* As the body temperature climbs, unexplained anxiety sets in. When the body temperature reaches 104°F to 105°F, the individual may feel a cold sensation in the trunk of the body, goose bumps, nausea, throbbing in the temples, and numbness in the extremities. Most people become incoherent after this stage. When body temperature reaches 105°F to 106°F, disorientation, loss of fine-motor control, and muscular weakness set in. If the temperature exceeds 106°F, serious neurologic injury and death may be imminent.

Heat stroke requires immediate emergency medical attention. Request help and get out of the sun. While you're waiting to be taken to the hospital's emergency room, your body should be sprayed with cool water and rubbed with cool towels. You also should be fanned and given plenty of cold liquids.

Q *What are the recommended guidelines for fluid replacement during prolonged aerobic exercise?*

A The main objective of fluid replacement during prolonged aerobic exercise is to maintain the blood volume so circulation and sweating can continue at normal levels. Adequate water replacement is the most important factor in preventing heat disorders. Drinking about 6 to 8 ounces of cool water every 15 to 20 minutes during exercise seems to be ideal to prevent dehydration. Cold fluids are absorbed more rapidly from the stomach.

Commercial fluid replacement solutions (e.g., Exceed, All-Sport, Gatorade) contain about 6% to 8% glucose, which seems to be optimal for fluid absorption and performance in most cases. Sugar does not become available to the muscles until about 30 minutes after drinking a glucose solution.

Drinks high in fructose or with a glucose concentration above 8% will slow down water absorption when exercising in the heat. Most soft drinks (cola, noncola) contain between 10% and 12% glucose, an amount that is too high for proper rehydration during exercise in the heat.

Commercially prepared sports drinks are recommended especially when exercise will be strenuous and carried out for more than an hour. For exercise lasting less than an hour, water is sufficient to replace fluid loss. The sports drinks that you select should be based on your personal preference. Try different drinks at 6% to 8% glucose concentration to see which drink you tolerate best and suits your taste as well.

During long-distance events researchers recommend that 50 to 60 grams of carbohydrate (200 to 240 calories) be consumed every hour. This is best accomplished by drinking 8 ounces of a 6% to 8% carbohydrate sports drink every 15 minutes. The percentage of the carbohydrate drink is determined by dividing the amount of carbohydrate, in grams, by the amount of fluid, in ml, and multiplying by 100. For example, 18 grams of carbohydrate in 240 ml (8 oz) of fluid yields a drink at 7.5% (18 ÷ 240 × 100).

Q *What precautions must a person take when exercising in the cold?*

A When exercising in the cold, the two factors to consider are frostbite and hypothermia (a breakdown in the body's ability to generate heat with a drop in temperature below 95°F). In contrast to hot and humid conditions, exercising in the cold usually does not threaten one's health because clothing for heat conservation can be selected and exercise itself increases the production of body heat.

Most people actually overdress for exercise in the cold. Because exercise increases body temperature, a moderate workout on a cold day makes you feel that it is 20-30° warmer than the actual temperature. Overdressing for exercise can make the clothes damp from excessive perspiration. The risk for hypothermia increases when a person is wet or not moving around sufficiently to increase body heat. Initial warning signs of hypothermia include shivering, loss of coordination, and difficulty in speaking. With a continued drop in body temperature, shivering

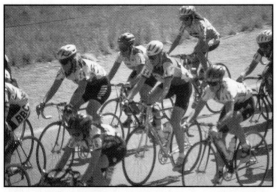

Fluid and carbohydrate replacement are essential during exercise of prolonged duration.

stops, the muscles weaken and stiffen, and the person experiences feelings of elation or intoxication and eventually loses consciousness. To prevent hypothermia, use common sense, dress properly, and be aware of environmental conditions.

The popular belief that exercising in cold temperatures (32°F and lower) freezes the lungs is false because the air is warmed properly in the air passages before it reaches the lungs. Cold is not what poses a threat. Rather, wind velocity is what affects the chill factor greatly.

For example, exercising at a temperature of 25°F with adequate clothing is not too cold, but if the wind is blowing at 25 miles per hour, the chill factor lowers the actual temperature to −5°F. This effect is even worse if a person is wet and exhausted. When windy, exercise (jog, cycle) against the wind on the way out and with the wind when you return.

Even though the lungs are under no risk when exercising in the cold, the face, head, hands, and feet should be protected, as they are subject to frostbite. Watch for signs of frostbite: numbness and discoloration. In cold temperatures about 30% of the body's heat is lost through the head's surface area if it is unprotected. A wool or synthetic cap, hood, or hat will help to hold in body heat. Mittens are better than gloves because they keep the fingers together, so the surface area from which to lose heat is less. Inner linings of synthetic material to wick (draw) moisture away from the skin are recommended.

Wearing several layers of lightweight clothing is preferable to wearing one single, thick layer because warm air is trapped between layers of clothes, enabling greater heat conservation. As body temperature increases, you can remove layers as necessary. For lengthy or long-distance workouts (cross-country skiing or long runs) take a small backpack to carry the clothing removed. You also can carry extra warm and dry clothes in case you stop exercising away from shelter. If you remain outdoors following exercise, added clothing and continuous body movement are essential.

The first layer of clothes should wick moisture away from the skin. Polypropylene, Capilene, or Thermax are recommended. Next, a layer of wool, dacron, or polyester fleece insulates well even when wet. Lycra tights or sweatpants help protect the legs. The outer layer should be waterproof, wind-resistant, and breathable. A synthetic material such as Gortex is best so moisture still can escape from the body. A ski or face mask helps protect the face. In extremely cold conditions any exposed skin, such as the nose, cheeks, or around the eyes, can be insulated with petroleum jelly.

SPECIAL CONSIDERATIONS FOR WOMEN

Q *What are the physiological differences between men and women as related to exercise?*

A Men and women have several basic differences that affect physical performance. On the average, men are about 3 to 4 inches taller and 25 to 30 pounds heavier. The average body fat in college males is about 12% to 16%, whereas in college females it is 22% to 26%.

Maximal oxygen uptake (aerobic capacity) is about 15% to 30% greater in men, primarily related to a higher hemoglobin concentration and the lower body fat content in men. The higher hemoglobin concentration allows men to carry a greater amount of oxygen during exercise, which is advantageous during aerobic events.

The quality of muscle in men and women is the same. Men, however, are stronger because they have a greater amount of muscle mass and a greater capacity for muscle hypertrophy, the *muscle's ability to increase in size*. The larger capacity for muscle hypertrophy is related to sex-specific hormones. Strength differences, nevertheless, are significantly less when taking into consideration body size and composition.

Men also have wider shoulders, longer extremities, and a 10% greater bone width, except for pelvic width. Notwithstanding all these gender differences in physiological characteristics, the two sexes respond to training in a similar way.

Q *If the potential for muscle hypertrophy in women is not as great, why do so many women body builders develop such heavy musculature?*

A The idea that strength training allows women to develop muscle hypertrophy to the same extent as men do is as false as the notion that playing basketball will turn women into giants. Masculinity and femininity are established by genetic inheritance, not by the amount of physical activity. Variations in the extent of masculinity and femininity are determined by individual differences in hormonal secretions of androgen, testosterone, estrogen, and progesterone. Women with a bigger-than-average build often are inclined to participate in sports because of their natural physical advantage. As a result, many women have associated participation in sports and strength training with large muscle size.

As the number of women who participate in sports has increased steadily during the last few years, the misconception that strength training in women leads to large increases in muscle size has abated somewhat. For example, per pound of body weight, women gymnasts are considered to be among the strongest athletes in the world. These athletes engage regularly in serious strength-training programs. Yet, female gymnasts have some of the most well-toned and graceful figures of all women. In recent years improved body appearance has become the rule rather than the exception for women who participate in strength-training programs. Some of the most attractive female movie stars also train with weights to improve their personal image. In his textbook *Weight Training for Life*, Dr. James Hesson pointed out that many beauty pageant participants engage in some sort of strength training program as they prepare for the pageant.[2] A survey at one state beauty pageant revealed that 86% of the participants (38 of 44 contestants) exercised with weights!

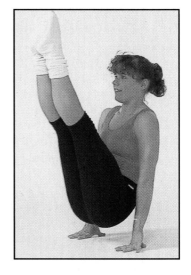

Contrary to some beliefs, high levels of strength do not lead to large muscle size in women.

At the same time, you may ask, "If weight training doesn't masculinize women, why do so many women body builders develop such heavy musculature?" In the sport of body building, the athletes follow intense training routines consisting of two or more hours of constant weight lifting with short rest intervals between sets. Many times body-building training routines call for back-to-back exercises using the same muscle groups. The objective of this type of training is to pump extra blood into the muscles, which makes the muscles appear much bigger than they really are in a resting condition. Based on the intensity and the length of the training session, the muscles can remain filled with blood and appear measurably larger for several hours after completing the training session. Therefore, in real life, these women are not as muscular as they seem when they are "pumped up" for a contest.

In the sport of body building, a big point of controversy is the use of anabolic steroids and human growth hormones, by women as well as men. Anabolic steroids are a *synthetic version of the male sex hormone testosterone, which promotes muscle development and hypertrophy.* These hormones produce detrimental and undesirable side effects, which some women deem tolerable (e.g., hypertension, fluid retention, decreased breast size, deepening of the voice, facial whiskers, and growth of body hair). Anabolic steroid use in general, except for medical reasons and when monitored carefully by a physician, can have serious health consequences.

Anabolic steroid use among women body builders is widespread. According to several sports medicine physicians and women body builders, about 80% of women body builders have used steroids. Furthermore, according to several women's track-and-field coaches, as many as 95% of women athletes in this sport around the world used anabolic steroids to remain competitive at the international level.

Undoubtedly women who take steroids will build heavy musculature, and, if they take the steroids long enough, will reveal masculinizing effects. As a result, the International Federation of Body Building instituted a mandatory steroid-testing program for women participating in the Miss Olympia contest. When drugs are not used to promote development, improved body image is the rule rather than the exception in women who participate in body building, strength training, and sports in general.

Q Does participation in exercise hinder menstruation?

A In some instances highly trained athletes develop amenorrhea, *stopping of menstruation*, during training and competition. This condition is seen most often in extremely lean women who also engage in sports that require strenuous physical effort over a sustained time. It is by no means irreversible. At present we do not know whether the condition is caused by physical stress or emotional stress related to high-intensity training, excessively low body fat, or other factors.

Although women on the average have a lower physical capacity during menstruation, women have broken Olympic and world records at all stages of the menstrual cycle. Menstruation should not keep a woman from participating in athletics, and it will not necessarily have a negative impact on performance.

Q Does exercise help relieve dysmenorrhea?

A Exercise has not been shown to either cure or aggravate *painful menstruation*, but it has been shown to help relieve menstrual cramps because it improves circulation to the uterus. Particularly, stretching exercises of the muscles in the pelvic region seem to reduce and prevent painful menstruation that is not the result of a disease.

Q Is exercising during pregnancy safe?

A Women should not forsake exercise during pregnancy. If anything, they should exercise to strengthen the body and prepare for delivery. Moderate exercise during pregnancy helps to prevent excessive weight gain and speed up recovery following birth. Pregnant women in American Indian tribes continue to do all of their difficult work chores up to the very day of delivery, and a few hours after the baby's birth they resume their normal activities. Women athletes have competed in sports during the early stages of pregnancy. The woman and her personal physician should make the final decision regarding her exercise program.

Stretching exercises are to be performed gently because hormonal changes during pregnancy increase the laxity of muscles and connective tissue. These changes facilitate delivery, but they also make women more susceptible to injuries during exercise. In 1994 the American College of Obstetricians and Gynecologists released an update of its guidelines for exercise during pregnancy.[3] Among the recommendations for pregnant women with no additional risk factors are:

1. Continue to exercise at a mild-to-moderate pace throughout the pregnancy, but decrease exercise intensity by about 25% from the prepregnancy program.

2. Exercise regularly a minimum of three times a week instead of doing occasional exercise bouts.

3. Pay attention to the body's signals of discomfort and distress. Stop exercise when tired. Never exercise to exhaustion. Stop if unusual symptoms arise, such as pain of any kind, cramping, nausea, bleeding, leaking of amniotic fluid, faintness, dizziness, palpitations, numbness in any part of the body, or decreased fetal activity.

4. After the first trimester avoid exercises that require you to lie on your back. This position can block blood flow to the uterus and the baby.

5. Do nonweight-bearing activities such as cycling, swimming, or water aerobics, which minimize the risk of injury and may allow continuation of exercise throughout pregnancy.

6. Avoid activities that could lead to a loss of balance or cause even mild trauma to the abdomen.

7. Take care to get proper nourishment. (Also, pregnancy requires approximately 300 extra calories per day.)

8. During the first three months in particular, avoid exercising in the heat. Wear clothing that allows for proper dissipation of heat and drink plenty of water.

Q *What is osteoporosis, and how can it be prevented?*

A Osteoporosis is *the softening, deterioration, or loss of total body bone.* Bones become so weak and brittle that the person is vulnerable to fractures, primarily of the hip, wrist, and spine. Osteoporosis is a preventable condition. It begins slowly in the third and fourth decades of life.

The importance of normal estrogen levels, adequate calcium intake, and physical activity cannot be overemphasized in maximizing bone density in young women and lowering the rate of bone loss later in life. All three factors are crucial in preventing osteoporosis. The absence of any one of these three factors leads to bone loss, for which the other two never compensate completely.

Prevention of osteoporosis should begin early in life by having enough calcium in the diet (RDA of 800 to 1,200 mg per day) and by participating in a lifetime exercise program. Also, vitamin D, which is necessary for optimal calcium absorption, may have to be supplemented. To further enhance calcium absorption and decrease calcium loss, alcohol, caffeine, and protein intake should be controlled; cigarettes should be eliminated; and an extremely high-fiber diet should be avoided. A list of selected foods and their respective calcium content is provided in Table 8.2. Weight-bearing exercises such as walking, jogging, and weight training are especially helpful. Not only do they tone up muscles, but they also produce stronger and thicker bones.

Prevailing research tells us that estrogen is the most important factor in preventing bone loss. Lumbar bone density in women with regular menstrual cycles exceeds that of women with a history of oligomenorrhea, *irregular cycles;* and amenorrhea (cessation of menstruation), interspaced with regular cycles. Furthermore, the lumbar density of these two groups of women is higher than that of women who never had regular cycles.

Women are especially susceptible to osteoporosis after menopause because the accompanying estrogen loss hastens the rate at which bone mass is broken down. Following menopause, every woman should consider hormone replacement therapy and discuss it with her physician. Women who have estrogen therapy do not lose bone mineral density at the rate that nontherapy women do. Neither exercise nor calcium supplementation will offset the damaging effects of lower estrogen levels.

Q *Do women have special iron needs?*

A Iron is a key element of hemoglobin in the blood, which carries oxygen from the lungs to all tissues of the body. The RDA of iron for adult women is 15 mg per day (10 mg for men).

TABLE 8.2 ❖ Low-Fat Calcium-Rich Foods

Food	Amount	Calcium (mg)	Calories	Calories from Fat
Beans, red kidney, cooked	1 cup	70	218	4%
Beet, greens, cooked	1/2 cup	72	13	—
Broccoli, cooked, drained	1 sm stalk	123	36	—
Burrito, bean	1	173	307	28%
Cottage cheese, 2% low-fat	1/2 cup	78	103	18%
Milk, nonfat, powdered	1 tbsp	52	27	1%
Milk, skim	1 cup	296	88	3%
Ice milk (vanilla)	1/2 cup	102	100	27%
Instant breakfast, whole milk	1 cup	301	280	26%
Kale, cooked, drained	1/2 cup	103	22	—
Okra, cooked, drained	1/2 cup	74	23	—
Shrimp, boiled	3 oz.	99	99	9%
Spinach, raw	1 cup	51	14	—
Yogurt, fruit	1 cup	345	231	8%
Yogurt, low-fat, plain	1 cup	271	160	20%

According to a survey by the U.S. Department of Agriculture, 19- to 50-year-old women in the United States consumed only 60% of the RDA for iron. People who do not have enough iron in the body can develop iron-deficiency anemia, in which the concentration of hemoglobin in the red blood cells is less than it should be.

Physically active women also may have a greater than average need for iron. Heavy training creates a demand for iron that is higher than the recommended intake because small amounts of iron are lost through sweat, urine, and stools. Mechanical trauma, caused by the pounding of the feet on the pavement during extensive jogging, also may lead to the destruction of iron-containing red blood cells.

Among female endurance athletes, a large percentage is reported to have iron deficiency. Blood ferritin levels, a measure of stored iron in the human body, should be checked frequently in women who participate in intense physical training.

The rates of iron absorption and iron loss vary from person to person. In most cases, though, people can get enough iron by eating more iron-rich foods such as beans, peas, green leafy vegetables, enriched grain products, egg yolk, fish, and lean meats. Although organ meats such as liver are especially good sources, they also are high in cholesterol. A list of foods high in iron content is given in Table 8.3.

NUTRITION AND WEIGHT CONTROL QUESTIONS

Q *What is the difference between a calorie and a kilocalorie (kcal)?*

A Calorie is *the unit of measure indicating the energy value of food and cost of physical activity*. Technically, a kilocalorie (kcal) or large calorie is *the amount of heat necessary to raise the temperature of 1 kilogram of water 1°C*. For simplification, people call it a calorie

TABLE 8.3 ❖ Iron-Rich Foods

Food	Amount	Iron (mg)	Calories	Cholesterol	Calories from Fat
Beans, red kidney, cooked	1 cup	4.4	218	0	4%
Beef, ground lean	3 oz.	3.0	186	81	48%
Beef, sirloin	3 oz.	2.5	329	77	74%
Beef, liver, fried	3 oz.	7.5	195	345	42%
Beet greens, cooked	1/2 cup	1.4	13	0	—
Broccoli, cooked, drained	1 sm stalk	1.1	36	0	—
Burrito, bean	1	2.4	307	14	28%
Egg, hard cooked	1	1.0	72	250	63%
Farina (Cream of Wheat), cooked	1/2 cup	6.0	51	0	—
Instant breakfast, whole milk	1 cup	8.0	280	33	26%
Peas, frozen, cooked, drained	1/2 cup	1.5	55	0	—
Shrimp, boiled	3 oz.	2.7	99	128	9%
Spinach, raw	1 cup	1.7	14	0	—
Vegetables, mixed, cooked	1 cup	2.4	116	0	—

rather than kcal. For example, if the caloric value of a food is 100 calories (kcal), the energy in this food could raise the temperature of 100 kilograms of water by 1°C.

Q *Does cooking affect the caloric content of food?*

A Cooking does not alter the caloric content of food significantly. The only exception is meat, in which broiling and barbecuing drain off some of the fat and decrease the caloric content. Frying, on the other hand, increases the caloric content of food significantly because of the large number of calories in the oil in which the food is fried.

Q *Is it true that calories don't count if I'm on a low-fat diet?*

A Some self-proclaimed nutrition experts would have you believe that the answer to the previous question is *yes*. A "nonfat" label

doesn't mean nonfattening when overindulging. Calories do count. And though most low-fat diets are also low in calories, you can't assume that all are. Eating too many calories, regardless of the source, results in weight gain. In addition, what you eat along with your carbohydrates make a difference. Salads and pasta are carbohydrate-rich, but many dressings and sauces that go along with them are not.

Q *Does heavy perspiration during exercise help a person lose weight?*

A Intense exercise, especially in warm or hot conditions, greatly enhances water loss (perspiration) from the body. You sweat off water, not fat. Without fluid replacement, a person can lose between 3 and 8 pounds of weight (water) per hour, depending on body size and ambient temperature. Once fluid is replaced after exercise, the weight is regained quickly. Fluids, however, should be replaced regularly

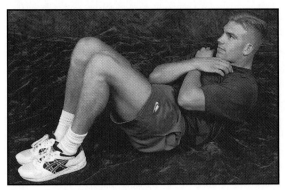
Spot-reducing does not work.

during exercise. As pointed out earlier, fluid replacement is crucial for optimal performance and proper heat balance.

Q Are rubberized sweatsuits and steam baths effective in losing weight?

A The answer to this question is simply *no*! When a person wears a sweatsuit or steps into a sauna, the weight lost is not fat but is merely a significant amount of water. Sure, it looks nice when you step on the scale immediately afterward, but this represents a false loss of weight. As soon as you replace body fluids, you gain back the weight quickly.

Wearing rubberized sweatsuits not only hastens the rate of body fluid loss — fluid that is vital during prolonged exercise — but at the same time raises the body's core temperature. This combination puts a person in danger of dehydration, which impairs cellular function and in extreme cases even can cause death.

Q Are mechanical vibrators useful in losing weight?

A Some people will try almost anything to lose weight as long as they can still over-indulge. These people can be deceived easily and often resort to quick fixes in an attempt to solve their weight problem. Mechanical vibrators are worthless in a weight-control program. Vibrating belts and turning rollers may feel good, but they require no effort whatsoever. A person

would have to vibrate continuously for 76 hours to lose the energy equivalent to 1 pound of fat! Fat cannot be "shaken off"; the body uses it as an energy substrate, and it is lost most efficiently by burning it in muscle tissue.

Q How detrimental is coffee to good health?

A Caffeine is a drug and as such can produce several undesirable side effects. Caffeine doses of more than 200 to 500 mg can cause an inordinately rapid heart rate, abnormal heart rhythms, a rise in blood pressure, higher body temperature, and oversecretion of gastric acids, leading to stomach problems. It also may have some link to birth defects in unborn children. It, too, may induce symptoms of anxiety, depression, nervousness, and dizziness. The caffeine content of various types of coffee ranges from 65 mg per 6 ounces for instant coffee to as high as 180 mg for drip coffee. Soft drinks, mainly colas, range in caffeine content from 30 mg to 60 mg per 12-ounce can.

Q Do athletes or individuals who train for long periods need a special diet?

A In general, athletes do not require special supplementation or any other special type of diet. Unless the diet is deficient in basic nutrients, no special, secret, or magic diet will help people perform better or develop faster as a result of what they eat. As long as the diet is balanced, based on a large variety of nutrients from the basic food groups, athletes do not require supplements. Even in strength training and body building, protein in excess of 20% of total daily caloric intake is not necessary.

The main difference between a sedentary person and a highly active individual is in the total number of calories required daily and the amount of carbohydrate intake during bouts of prolonged physical activity. During training, people consume more calories because of the greater energy expenditure required as a result of intense physical training.

A regular diet should be altered to include about 70% carbohydrates (carbohydrate loading) during several days of heavy aerobic training or when a person is going to participate in a long-distance event of more than 90 minutes (marathons, triathlons, road cycling races). For events shorter than 90 minutes, carbohydrate loading does not seem to enhance performance.

EXERCISE AND AGING

Q *What about exercise programs for older adults?*

A Unlike any prior time in American history, the elderly population constitutes the fastest growing segment. In 1880 less than 3% of the total population, fewer than 2 million people, was older than 65. By 1980 the elderly population had reached approximately 25 million, more than 11.3% of the population. According to estimates, the elderly will make up more than 20% of the total population by the year 2035.

Older adults have been neglected when developing fitness programs, even though, fitness is just as important for older people as it is for young people. Although much research remains to be done in this area, studies indicate that older individuals who are physically fit also enjoy better health and quality of life.

The main objective of fitness programs for older adults should be to help them improve their functional health status. This implies the ability to maintain independent living status and avoid disability. A committee of the American Alliance of Health, Physical Education, Recreation and Dance (AAHPERD) has defined functional fitness for older adults as *the physical capacity of the individual to meet ordinary and unexpected demands of daily life safely and effectively.*[4] This definition clearly indicates the need for fitness programs that relate closely to activities this population normally encounters. The AAHPERD committee encourages participation in programs that will help develop cardiorespiratory endurance, localized muscular endurance, muscular flexibility, agility and balance, and motor coordination. A copy of the battery of fitness tests for older adults can be obtained from AAHPERD, Reston, Virginia.

Q *What is the relationship between aging and physical work capacity?*

A Although previous research studies have documented declines in physiological functioning and motor capacity as a result of aging, no hard evidence at present proves that declines in physical work capacity are related primarily to the aging process. Lack of physical activity — a common phenomenon seen in our society as people age — may be accompanied by decreases in physical work capacity that are greater by far than the effects of aging itself.

Data on individuals who have taken part in systematic physical activity throughout life indicate that these groups of people maintain a higher level of functional capacity and do not experience the typical declines in later years. From a functional point of view, the typical sedentary American is about 25 years older than his or her chronological age indicates. Thus, an active 60-year-old person can have a work capacity similar to that of a sedentary 35-year-old.

Unfortunately, unhealthy behaviors precipitate premature aging. For sedentary people, productive life ends at about age 60. Most of these

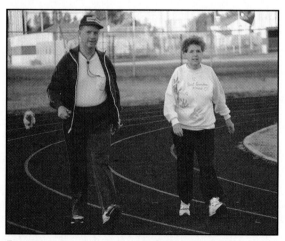

Exercise enhances quality of life and longevity.

people hope to live to be 65 or 70 and often must cope with serious physical ailments. These people stop living at age 60 but choose to be buried at age 70 (see Figure 8.2)!

Scientists believe a healthy lifestyle allows people to live a vibrant life — a physically, intellectually, emotionally, socially active, and functionally independent existence — to age 95. When death comes to active people, it usually is rather quick and not as a result of prolonged illness (see Figure 8.2). Such are the rewards of a wellness way of life.

Q *Do older adults respond to physical training?*

A The trainability of elderly men and women alike and the effectiveness of physical activity for enhancing health have been demonstrated in prior research. Older adults who increase their level of physical activity go through significant changes in cardiorespiratory endurance, strength, and flexibility. The extent of the changes depends on their initial fitness level and the types of activities selected for their training (walking, cycling, strength training, and so on).

Improvements in maximal oxygen uptake in older adults are similar to those of younger people, although older people seem to require a longer training period to achieve these changes. Declines in cardiorespiratory endurance (maximal oxygen uptake) per decade of life after age 25 seem to be about 9% for sedentary adults and 5% or less in active people.

Results of a study on the effects of aging on the cardiorespiratory system of male exercisers versus nonexercisers showed that the maximal oxygen uptake of regular exercisers was almost twice that of the nonexercisers.[5] The study revealed a decline in maximal oxygen uptake between the ages 50 and 68 of only 13% in the active group, compared to 41% in the inactive group. These changes indicate that about one-third of the loss in maximal oxygen uptake results from aging and two-thirds from inactivity. Blood pressure, heart rate, and body weight also were remarkably better in the exercising group.

Older adults can increase their strength levels, too, but the amount of muscle hypertrophy achieved decreases with age. Strength gains close to 200% have been found in previously inactive adults over age 90. In terms of body composition, inactive adults continue to gain body fat after age 60 despite the tendency toward lower body weight.

Older adults who wish to initiate or continue an exercise program are encouraged strongly to have a complete medical exam, including a stress electrocardiogram test (see Chapter 7). Recommended activities for older adults include calisthenics,

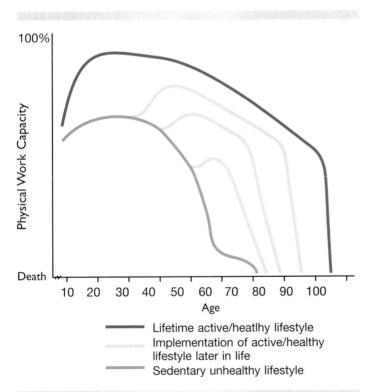

FIGURE 8.2 ❖ Relationship between physical work capacity, aging, and lifestyle habits.

walking, jogging, swimming, cycling, and water aerobics.

Older people should avoid isometric and other intense weight-training exercises. Activities that require all-out effort or require participants to hold their breath (valsalva maneuver) tend to lessen blood flow to the heart and cause a significant increase in blood pressure and load on the heart. Older adults should participate in activities that require continuous and rhythmic muscular activity (about 50% to 70% of functional capacity) and strength training with light weights. These activities do not cause large increases in blood pressure or place an intense overload on the heart.

As illustrated in Figure 8.2, physical fitness or physical work capacity can be increased at any age. Complete benefits of a healthy lifestyle, nonetheless, are best attained by starting early in life.

FITNESS/WELLNESS CONSUMER ISSUES

Q *How can I protect myself from fitness/wellness quackery and fraud?*

A The rapid growth in fitness and wellness programs during the last three decades has spurred the promotion of fraudulent products that deceive consumers into adopting "miraculous," quick, and easy ways toward total well-being. Quackery and fraud have been defined as the *conscious promotion of unproven claims for profit.*

Today's market is saturated with "special" foods, diets, supplements, pills, cures, equipment, books, and videos that promise quick, dramatic results. Advertisements for these products often are based on testimonials, unproven claims, secret research, half-truths, and quick-fix statements that the uneducated consumer wants to hear. In the meantime, the organization or enterprise making the claims stands to reap a large profit from the consumers' willingness to pay for astonishing and spectacular solutions to problems related to their unhealthy lifestyle.

Television, magazine, and newspaper advertisements are not necessarily reliable. For instance, one piece of equipment sold through television and newspaper advertisements promised to "bust the gut" through 5 minutes of daily exercise that appeared to target the abdominal muscle group. This piece of equipment consisted of a metal spring attached to the feet on one end and held in the hands on the other end. According to handling and shipping distributors, the equipment was "selling like hotcakes," and companies could barely keep up with the consumer's demands.

Three problems became apparent to the educated consumer. First, there is no such thing as spot-reducing; therefore, the claims could not be true. Second, 5 minutes of daily exercise burn hardly any calories and, therefore, have no effect on weight loss. Third, the intended abdominal (gut) muscles were not really involved during the exercise. The exercise engaged mostly the gluteal and lower back muscles. This piece of equipment now can be found at garage sales for about a tenth of its original cost!

Although people in the United States tend to firmly believe in the benefits of physical activity and positive lifestyle habits as a means to promote better health, most people do not reap these benefits because they simply do not know how to put into practice a sound fitness and wellness program that will give them the results they want. Unfortunately, many uneducated wellness consumers are targets of deception by organizations making fraudulent claims for their products.

Even though deceit is all around us, we can protect ourselves from consumer fraud. The first step is *education.* You have to be an informed consumer of the product you intend to purchase. If you do not have or cannot find the answers, seek the advice of a reputable professional. Ask someone who understands the product but does not stand to profit from the transaction. As examples, a physical educator or an exercise physiologist can advise you regarding exercise equipment; a registered dietitian can provide information on nutrition and weight-control programs; a physician can offer advice on treatment modalities. Also, be alert to those who bill themselves as "experts." Look for qualifications, degrees, professional experience, certifications, reputation.

Another clue to possible fraud is that if it sounds too good to be true, it probably is. Quick-fix, miraculous, special, secret, mail orders only, money-back guarantee, and testimonials often are announced in advertisements of fraudulent promotions. When claims are made, ask where the claims are published. Newspapers, magazines, and trade books are apt to be unreliable sources of information. Refereed scientific journals are the most reliable sources of information. When a researcher submits information for publication in a refereed journal, at least two qualified and reputable professionals in the field conduct blind reviews of the manuscript. A blind review means the author does not know who will review the manuscript and the reviewers do not know who submitted the manuscript. Acceptance for publication is based on this input and relevant changes.

If you have questions or concerns about a health product, you may write to the National Council Against Health Fraud (NCAHF), P.O. Box 1276, Loma Linda, CA 92354. The purpose of this organization is to monitor deceitful advertising, investigate complaints, and offer the public information regarding fraudulent health claims.

Q *What guidelines should I follow when looking for a reputable health-fitness facility?*

A As you follow a lifetime wellness program, you may want to consider joining a health/fitness facility. Or, if you have mastered the contents of this book and your choice of fitness activity is one you can pursue on your own (walking, jogging, cycling), you may not need to join a health club. Barring injuries, you may continue your exercise program outside the walls of a health club for the rest of your life. You also can conduct strength-training and stretching programs within the walls of your own home (see Chapters 3, 4 and Appendices B, C, and D).

To stay up to date on fitness and wellness developments, you probably should buy a reputable and updated fitness/wellness book every 4 to 5 years. You also might subscribe to a credible health, fitness, nutrition, or wellness newsletter (see Table 8.4) to stay current.

If you are contemplating membership in a fitness facility:

❖ Examine all exercise options in your community: health clubs/spas, YMCAs, gyms, colleges, schools, community centers, senior centers, and the like.

❖ Check to see if the facility's atmosphere is pleasurable and nonthreatening to you. Will you feel comfortable with the instructors and other people who go there? Is it clean and well kept up? If the answer is no, this may not be the right place for you.

❖ Analyze costs versus facilities, equipment, and programs. Take a look at your personal budget. Will you really use the facility? Will you exercise there regularly? Many people obtain memberships and allow dues to be withdrawn automatically from a local bank account, yet seldom attend the fitness center.

❖ Find out what types of facilities are available: running track, basketball/tennis/racquetball courts, aerobic exercise room, strength-training room, pool, locker rooms, saunas, hot tubs, handicapped access, and so on.

❖ Check the aerobic and strength-training equipment available. Does the facility have treadmills, bicycle ergometers, Stair Masters, cross-country skiing simulators, free weights, Universal Gym, Nautilus? Make sure the facilities and equipment meet your activity interests.

❖ Consider the location. Is the facility close, or do you have to travel several miles to get there? Distance often discourages participation.

❖ Check on times the facility is accessible. Is it open during your preferred exercise time (for example, early morning or late evening)?

❖ Work out at the facility several times before becoming a member. Are people standing in line to use the equipment, or is it readily available during your exercise time?

❖ Inquire about the instructors' qualifications. Do the fitness instructors have college degrees or professional certifications from organizations such as the American College of Sports Medicine (ACSM) or the International Dance Exercise Association (IDEA)? These organizations have rigorous standards to ensure professional preparation and quality of instruction.

❖ Consider the approach to fitness (including all health-related components of fitness). Is it well-rounded? Do the instructors spend time with members, or do members have to seek them out constantly for help and instruction?

❖ Ask about supplementary services. Does the facility provide or contract out for regular health and fitness assessments (cardiorespiratory endurance, body composition, blood pressure, blood chemistry analysis)? Are wellness seminars (nutrition, weight control, stress management) offered? Do these have hidden costs?

Q *What factors should I consider prior to purchasing exercise equipment?*

A The first question you need to ask yourself is: Do I really need this piece of equipment? Most people buy on impulse because of television advertisements or because a salesperson convinced them that it is a great piece of equipment that will do wonders for their health and fitness. If marketing claims seem too good to be true, they probably are. With some creativity, you can implement an excellent and comprehensive exercise program with little, if any, equipment (see Chapters 3 and 4).

Many people buy expensive equipment only to find they really do not enjoy that mode of activity. They do not remain regular users. Stationary bicycles (lower body only) and rowing ergometers were among the most popular pieces of equipment in the 1980s. Most of them now are seldom used and have become "fitness furniture" somewhere in the basement.

Exercise equipment does have its value for people who prefer to exercise indoors, especially during the winter months. It supports some people's motivation and adherence to exercise. The convenience of having equipment at home also allows for flexible scheduling. You can exercise before or after work or while you watch your favorite television show.

If you are going to purchase equipment, the best recommendation is to actually try it out several times before buying it. Ask yourself several questions: Did you enjoy the workout? Is the unit comfortable? Are you too short, tall, or heavy for it? Is it stable, sturdy, and strong? Do you have to assemble the machine? If so, how difficult is it to put together? How durable is it? Ask for references — people or clubs that have used the equipment extensively. Are they satisfied? Have they enjoyed the activity (the equipment)? Talk with professionals at colleges, sportsmedicine clinics, or health clubs.

TABLE 8.4 ❖ Reliable Sources of Health, Fitness, Wellness, and Nutrition Information

Newsletter	Approx. Yearly Issues	Annual Cost
Consumer Reports Health Letter P.O. Box 56356 Boulder, CO 80323–2148	12	$24
Executive Health's Good Health Report P.O. Box 8880 Chapel Hill, NC 27515	12	$34
Tufts University Diet & Nutrition Letter P.O. Box 57857 Boulder, CO 80322–7857	12	$20
University of California Berkeley Wellness Letter P.O. Box 420148 Palm Coast, FL 32142	12	$20

Another consideration is to look at used units for signs of wear and tear. Quality is important. Cheaper brands may not be durable, so your investment would be wasted.

Finally, watch out for expensive gadgets. Monitors that provide exercise heart rate, work output, caloric expenditure, speed, grade, and distance may help motivate you, but they are expensive, need repairs, and do not enhance the actual fitness benefits of the workout. Look at maintenance costs and check for service personnel in your community.

WHAT'S NEXT?

The objective of this book is to provide you with the information necessary to implement your personal healthy lifestyle program. Your activities over the last few weeks or months may have helped you develop positive habits that you should try to carry on throughout life.

Now that you are about to finish this course, the real challenge will be a lifetime commitment to fitness and wellness. Adhering to the program in a structured setting is a lot easier. Fitness and wellness is a continual process. As you proceed with the program, keep in mind that the greatest benefit is a higher quality of life.

Most people who adopt a wellness way of life recognize this new quality after only a few weeks into the program. In some instances, especially individuals who led a poor lifestyle for a long time, establishing positive habits and gaining feelings of well-being might take a few

A wellness way of life

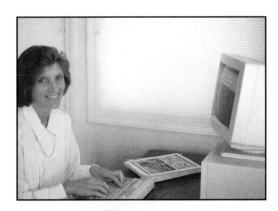

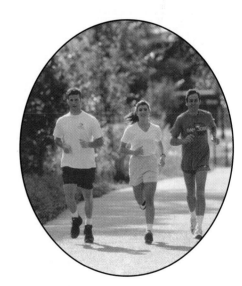

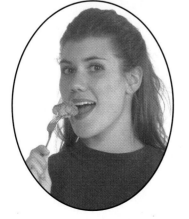

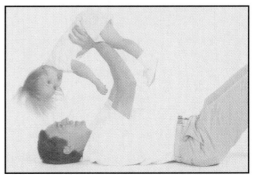

months. In the end, however, everyone who applies the principles of fitness and wellness will reap the desired benefits.

Being diligent and taking control of yourself will provide you a better, happier, healthier, and more productive life. Be sure to maintain a program based on your needs and what you enjoy doing most. Such practice will make the journey easier and more fun along the way. Once you reach the top, you will know there is no looking back. If you don't get there, you won't know what it's like. Improving the quality and longevity of your life is now in your hands. This will require persistence and commitment, but only *you can take control of your lifestyle and thereby reap the benefits of wellness.*

NOTES

1. R. S. Paffenbarger, Jr., R. T. Hyde, A. L. Wing, and C. H. Steinmetz. "A Natural History of Athleticism and Cardiovascular Health." *Journal of the American Medical Association*, 252 (1984), 491-495.

2. J. L. Hesson. *Weight Training for Life* (Englewood, CO: Morton Publishing, 1991).

3. American College of Obstetricians and Gynecologists, *Guidelines for Exercise During Pregnancy*, 1994.

4. W. H. Osness, M. Adrian, B. Clark, W. Hoeger, D. Raab, and R. Wiswell, *Functional Fitness Assessment for Adults Over 60 Years*. (Reston, VA: American Alliance for Health, Physical Education, Recreation, and Dance, 1990).

5. F. W. Kash, J. L. Boyer, S. P. Van Camp, L. S. Verity, and J. P. Wallace. "The Effect of Physical Activity on Aerobic Power in Older Men (A Longitudinal Study)," *The Physician and Sports Medicine*, 18:4 (1990), 73–83.

Pre- and Post-Fitness Profiles

Personal Fitness Profile: Pre-Test

Date: _____ Course: _____ Section: _____

Name: _____ Age: _____ Male or Female: M / F

Body Weight: _____ . _____

Fitness Component	Test Data	Test Results	Fitness Classification	Fitness Goal
Cardiorespiratory Endurance 1.5-Mile Run	Time _____ : _____	$VO_{2 max.}$ _____ . _____	_____	$VO_{2 max.}$ _____ . _____
1.0-Mile Walk	Time _____ : _____ Heart Rate _____	 $VO_{2 max.}$ _____ . _____	 _____	 $VO_{2 max.}$ _____ . _____
Muscular Strength / Endurance	Reps	Percentile		
Bench Jumps	_____	_____	_____	_____
Chair Dips / Mod. Push-Ups	_____	_____	_____	_____
Abdominal Crunches	_____	_____	_____	_____
Average Percentile		_____		
Muscular Flexibility	Inches	Percentile		
Modified Sit-and-Reach	_____	_____	_____	_____
Body Rotation (R/L)	_____	_____	_____	_____
Average Percentile		_____		
Body Composition	mm			
Chest / Triceps	_____			
Abdominal / Suprailium	_____			
Thigh	_____			
Sum of Skinfolds	_____			
Percent Body Fat		_____	_____	_____
Lean Body Mass (lbs.)		_____		_____

_____   _____   _____
Student Signature   Instructor Signature   Date

FIGURE A.1 ❖ Personal fitness profile: Pre-test.

Personal Fitness Profile: Post-Test

Date: _____ Course: _____ Section: _____

Name: _____ Age: _____ Male or Female: M / F

Body Weight: _____ . _____

Fitness Component	Test Data	Test Results	Fitness Classification
Cardiorespiratory Endurance **1.5-Mile Run**	Time _____ : _____	VO$_2$ max. _____ . _____	_____
1.0-Mile Walk	Time _____ : _____		
	Heart Rate _____	VO$_2$ max. _____ . _____	_____
Muscular Strength / Endurance	Reps	Percentile	
Bench Jumps	_____	_____	_____
Chair Dips / Mod. Push-Ups	_____	_____	_____
Abdominal Crunches	_____	_____	_____
Average Percentile	_____	_____	_____
Muscular Flexibility	Inches	Percentile	
Modified Sit-and-Reach	_____	_____	_____
Body Rotation (R/L)	_____	_____	_____
Average Percentile	_____	_____	_____
Body Composition	mm		
Chest / Triceps	_____		
Abdominal / Suprailium	_____		
Thigh	_____		
Sum of Skinfolds	_____		
Percent Body Fat	_____	_____	_____
Lean Body Mass (lbs.)	_____	_____	_____

Student Signature   Instructor Signature   Date

FIGURE A.2 ❖ Personal fitness profile: Post-test.

FITNESS PROFILE

Based on the textbook Fitness and Wellness
by Werner W.K. Hoeger and Sharon A. Hoeger
Morton Publishing Company
Englewood, Colorado

James Doe   Course: PE 114 Fitness Foundations
Age: 18   Section: 01
Gender: M   Instructor: Werner Hoeger

Test Item	Most Recent Test 09-22-1995	Current Test 12-14-1995	Current Fitness Rating	Percent Change
Cardiovascular Endurance (1.5-mile run test)	39.8 ml/kg/min	45.8 ml/kg/min	Good	+15
Muscular Endurance	37 %tile	60 %tile	Average	
Number of bench jumps	48 reps - 30 %tile	56 reps - 60 %tile	Average	+17
Number of chair dips	27 reps - 60 %tile	32 reps - 80 %tile	Good	+19
Number of crunches	24 reps - 20 %tile	27 reps - 40 %tile	Fair	+13
Muscular Flexibility	50 %tile	50 %tile	Average	
Sit and reach	16.5 in - 70 %tile	17.5 in - 70 %tile	Good	+6
Right body rotation	15.5 in - 30 %tile	17.0 in - 30 %tile	Fair	+10
Body Composition				
Percent body fat	23.7 %	21.4 %	Overweight	-10
Recommended percent body fat		20.0 %		
Body weight	175.0 lbs	170.5 lbs		
Recommended body weight		167.5 lbs		

*Computer software is available from Morton Publishing Company, Englewood, Colorado.

FIGURE A.3 ❖ Personal fitness profile: Pre-/Post-test.

Strength-Training Exercises Without Weights

EXERCISE 1   Step-Up

Action: Step up and down using a box or chair approximately twelve to fifteen inches high. Conduct one set using the same leg each time you go up and then conduct a second set using the other leg. You could also alternate legs on each step-up cycle. You may increase the resistance by holding a child or some other object in your arms (hold the child or object close to the body to avoid increased strain in the lower back).

Muscles Developed: Gluteal muscles, quadriceps, gastrocnemius, and soleus.

EXERCISE 2   High-Jumper

Action: Start with the knees bent at approximately 150° and jump as high as you can, raising both arms simultaneously.

Muscles Developed: Gluteal muscles, quadriceps, gastrocnemius, and soleus.

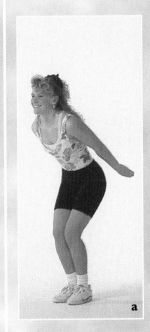

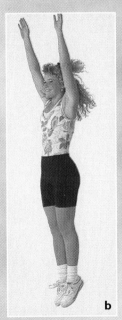

a   b

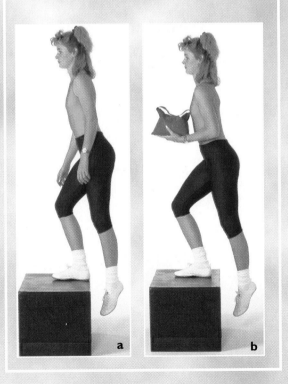

a   b

Photographs for Exercises 11, 14, 15, 16, and 17 are courtesy of Universal Gym® Equipment, Inc., 930 27th Avenue, S.W., Cedar Rapids, IA 52406. Photographs for Exercises 12 and 13 are courtesy of Nautilus®, a registered trademark of Nautilus® Sports/Medical Industries, Inc., P.O. Box 809014, Dallas, TX 75380-9014.

Push-Up

Action: Maintaining your body as straight as possible, flex the elbows, lowering the body until you almost touch the floor, then raise yourself back up to the starting position. If you are unable to perform the push-up as indicated, you can decrease the resistance by supporting the lower body with the knees rather than the feet (see illustration c) or using an incline plane and supporting your hands at a higher point than the floor (see illustration d). If you wish to increase the resistance, have someone else add resistance to your shoulders as you are coming back up (see illustration e).

Muscles Developed: Triceps, deltoid, pectoralis major, erector spinae, and abdominals.

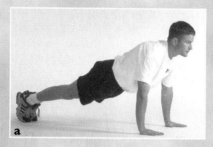

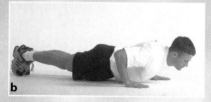

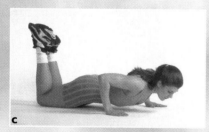

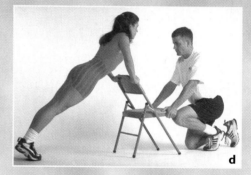

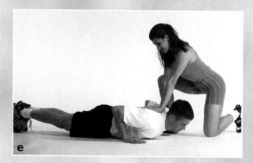

EXERCISE 4

Abdominal Crunch and Abdominal Curl-Up

Action: Start with your head and shoulders off the floor, arms crossed on your chest, and knees slightly bent (the greater the flexion of the knee, the more difficult the curl-up). Now curl up to about 30° (abdominal crunch — see illustration b) or curl all the way up (abdominal curl-up), then return to the starting position without letting the head or shoulders touch the floor, or allowing the hips to come off the floor. If you allow the hips to raise off the floor and the head and shoulders to touch the floor, you will most likely "swing up" on the next sit-up, which minimizes the work of the abdominal muscles. If you cannot curl up with the arms on the chest, place the hands by the side of the hips or even help yourself up by holding on to your thighs (illustrations d and e). Do not perform the sit-up exercise with your legs completely extended, as this will cause strain on the lower back.

Muscles Developed: Abdominal muscles (crunch) and hip flexors (complete curl-up).

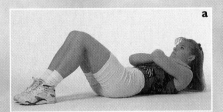
a

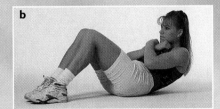
b

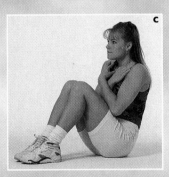
c

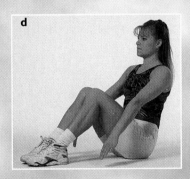
d

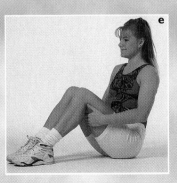
e

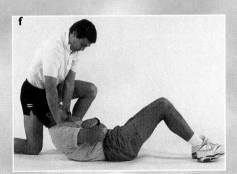
f

EXERCISE 5

Leg Curl

Action: Lie on the floor face down. Cross the right ankle over the left heel. Apply resistance with your right foot, while you bring the left foot up to 90° at the knee joint. (Apply enough resistance so that the left foot can only be brought up slowly.) Repeat the exercise, crossing the left ankle over the right heel.

Muscles Developed: Hamstrings (and quadriceps).

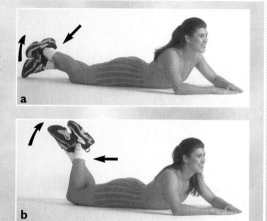

EXERCISE 6

Modified Dip

Action: Place your hands and feet on opposite chairs (make sure that the chairs are well stabilized). Dip down at least to a 90° angle at the elbow joint, then return to the initial position. To increase the resistance, have someone else hold you down by the shoulders on the way up (see illustration c).

Muscles Developed: Triceps, deltoid, and pectoralis major.

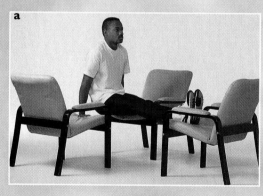

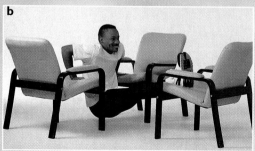

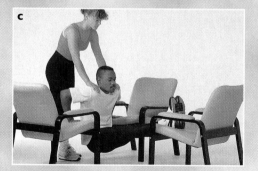

EXERCISE 7

Pull-Up

Action: Suspend yourself from a bar with a pronated grip (thumbs in). Pull your body up until your chin is above the bar, then lower the body slowly to the starting position. If you are unable to perform the pull-up as described, either have a partner hold your feet to push off and facilitate the movement upward (illustrations c and d) or use a lower bar and support your feet on the floor (illustration e).

Muscles Developed: Biceps, brachioradialis, brachialis, trapezius, and latissimus dorsi.

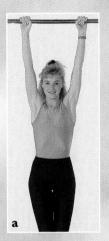

a

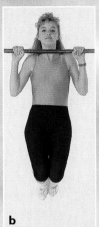

b

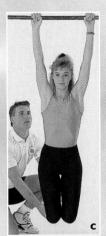

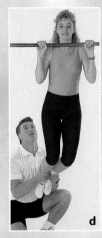

c

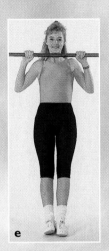

d

e

EXERCISE 8

Arm Curl

Action: Using a palms-up grip, start with the arm completely extended, and with the aid of a sandbag or bucket filled (as needed) with sand or rocks, curl up as far as possible, then return to the initial position. Repeat the exercise with the other arm.

Muscles Developed: Biceps, brachioradialis, and brachialis.

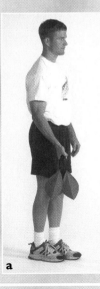

a

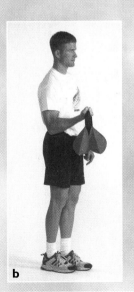

b

EXERCISE 9 — Heel Raise

Action: From a standing position with feet flat on the floor, raise and lower your body weight by moving at the ankle joint only (for added resistance, have someone else hold your shoulders down as you perform the exercise).

Muscles Developed: Gastrocnemius and soleus.

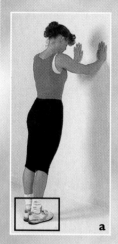
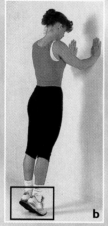

a   b

EXERCISE 10 — Leg Abduction and Adduction

Action: Both participants sit on the floor. The subject on the left places the feet on the inside of the other participant's feet. Simultaneously, the subject on the left presses the legs laterally (to the outside — abduction), while the subject on the right presses the legs medially (adduction). Hold the contraction for five to ten seconds. Repeat the exercise at all three angles, and then reverse the pressing sequence. The subject on the left places the feet on the outside and presses inward, while the subject on the right presses outward.

Muscles Developed: Hip abductors (rectus femoris, sartori, gluteus medius and minimus), and adductors (pectineus, gracilis, adductor magnus, adductor longus, and adductor brevis).

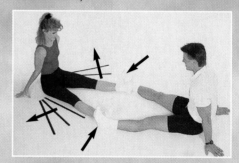

Strength-Training Exercises With Weights

EXERCISE 11 — Arm Curl

Action: Use a supinated or palms-up grip, and start with the arms almost completely extended. Now curl up as far as possible, then return to the starting position.

Muscles Developed: Biceps, brachioradialis, and brachialis.

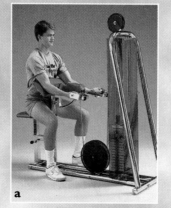
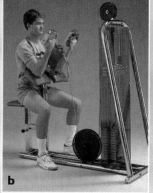

a   b

EXERCISE
12

Bench Press

Action: Lie down on the bench with the head by the weight stack, the bench press bar above the chest, and place the feet on the bench. Grasp the bar handles and press upward until the arms are completely extended, then return to the original position. Do not arch the back during this exercise.

Muscles Developed: Pectoralis major, triceps, and deltoid.

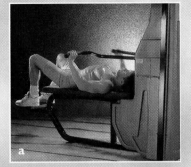
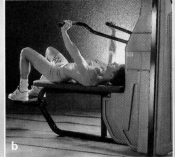

EXERCISE
13

Abdominal Crunch

Action Sit in an upright position and grasp the handles over your shoulders and crunch forward. Slowly return to the original position.

Muscles Developed Abdominals.

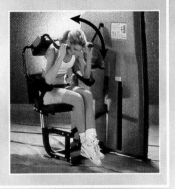

EXERCISE
14

Leg Extension

Action: Sit in an upright position with the feet under the padded bar and grasp the handles at the sides. Extend the legs until they are completely straight, then return to the starting position.

Muscles Developed: Quadriceps.

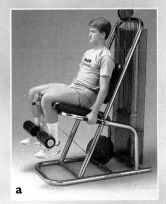
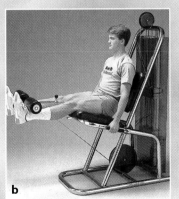

EXERCISE
15

Leg Curl

Action: Lie with the face down on the bench, legs straight, and place the back of the feet under the padded bar. Curl up to at least 90°, and return to the original position.

Muscles Developed: Hamstrings.

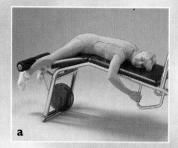

a

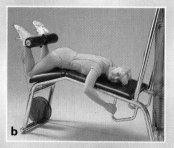

b

EXERCISE
16

Lat Pull-Down

Action: Start from a sitting position, and hold the exercise bar with a wide grip. Pull the bar down until it touches the base of the neck, then return to the starting position.

Muscles Developed: Latissimus dorsi, pectoralis major, and biceps.

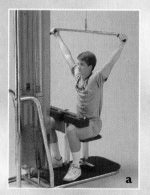

a

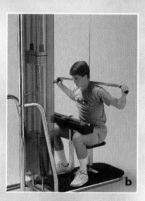

b

EXERCISE
17

Heel Raise

Action: Start with your feet either flat on the floor or the front of the feet on an elevated block, then raise and lower yourself by moving at the ankle joint only. If additional resistance is needed, you can use a squat strength-training machine.

Muscles Developed: Gastrocnemius and soleus.

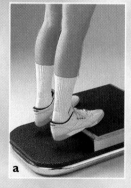

a

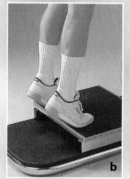

b

Flexibility Exercises

EXERCISE 18 — Lateral Head Tilt

Action: Slowly and gently tilt the head laterally. Repeat several times to each side.

Areas Stretched: Neck flexors and extensors and ligaments of the cervical spine.

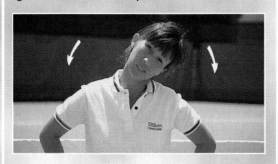

EXERCISE 19 — Arm Circles

Action: Gently circle your arms all the way around. Conduct the exercise in both directions.

Areas Stretched: Shoulder muscles and ligaments.

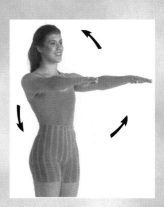

EXERCISE 20 — Side Stretch

Action: Stand straight up, feet separated to shoulder width, and place your hands on your waist. Now move the upper body to one side and hold the final stretch for a few seconds. Repeat on the other side.

Areas Stretched: Muscles and ligaments in the pelvic region.

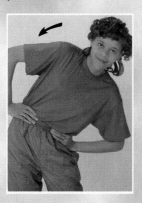

EXERCISE 21 — Body Rotation

Action: Place your arms slightly away from your body and rotate the trunk as far as possible, holding the final position for several seconds. Conduct the exercise for both the right and left sides of the body. You can also perform this exercise by standing about two feet away from the wall (back toward the wall), and then rotate the trunk, placing the hands against the wall.

Areas Stretched: Hip, abdominal, chest, back, neck, and shoulder muscles; hip and spinal ligaments.

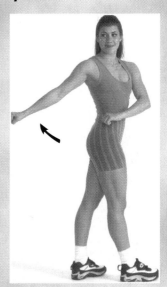

EXERCISE 22   Chest Stretch

Action: Kneel down behind a chair and place both hands on the back of the chair. Gradually push your chest downward and hold for a few seconds.

Areas Stretched: Chest (pectoral) muscles and shoulder ligaments.

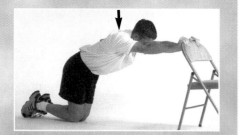

EXERCISE 23   Shoulder Hyperextension Stretch

Action: Have a partner grasp your arms from behind by the wrists and slowly push them upward. Hold the final position for a few seconds.

Areas Stretched: Deltoid and pectoral muscles, and ligaments of the shoulder joint.

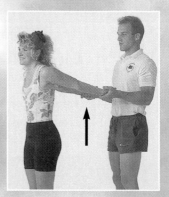

EXERCISE 24   Shoulder Rotation Stretch

Action: With the aid of surgical tubing or an aluminum or wood stick, place the tubing or stick behind your back and grasp the two ends using a reverse (thumbs-out) grip. Slowly bring the tubing or stick over your head, keeping the elbows straight. Repeat several times (bring the hands closer together for additional stretch).

Areas Stretched: Deltoid, latissimus dorsi, and pectoral muscles; shoulder ligaments.

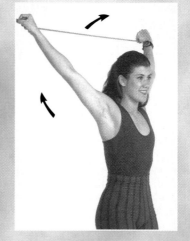

EXERCISE 25   Quad Stretch

Action: Lie on your side and move one foot back by flexing the knee. Grasp the front of the ankle and pull the ankle toward the gluteal region. Hold for several seconds. Repeat with the other leg.

Areas Stretched: Quadriceps muscle, and knee and ankle ligaments.

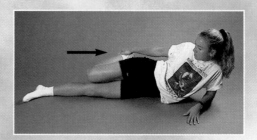

EXERCISE 26 — Heel Cord Stretch

Action: Assume a push-up position, then bend one knee and stretch the opposite heel cord. Hold the stretched position for a few seconds. Alternate legs. You may also perform this exercise leaning against a wall or standing at the edge of a step, then stretch the heel downward.

Areas Stretched: Heel cord (Achilles tendon), gastrocnemius, and soleus muscles.

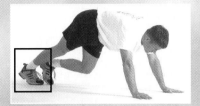

EXERCISE 27 — Adductor Stretch

Action: Stand with your feet about twice shoulder width and place your hands slightly above the knee. Flex one knee and slowly go down as far as possible, holding the final position for a few seconds. Repeat with the other leg.

Areas Stretched: Hip adductor muscles.

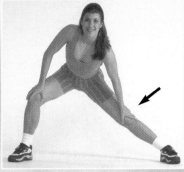

EXERCISE 28 — Sitting Adductor Stretch

Action: Sit on the floor and bring your feet in close to you, allowing the soles of the feet to touch each other. Now place your forearms (or elbows) on the inner part of the thigh and push the legs downward, holding the final stretch for several seconds.

Areas Stretched: Hip adductor muscles.

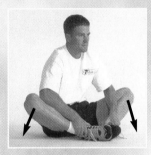

EXERCISE 29 — Sit-and-Reach Stretch

Action: Sit on the floor with legs together and gradually reach forward as far as possible. Hold the final position for a few seconds. This exercise may also be performed with the legs separated, reaching to each side as well as to the middle.

Areas Stretched: Hamstrings and lower back muscles, and lumbar spine ligaments.

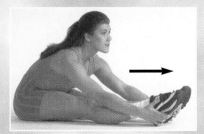

EXERCISE 30 — Triceps Stretch

Action: Place the right hand behind your neck. Grasp the right arm above the elbow with the left hand. Gently pull the elbow backward. Repeat the exercise with the opposite arm.

Areas Stretched: Back of upper arm (triceps muscle) and shoulder joint.

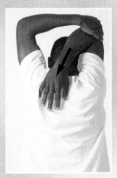

Exercises for the Prevention and Rehabilitation of Low Back Pain

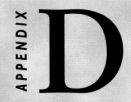

EXERCISE 31 — Single-Knee to Chest Stretch

Action: Lie down flat on the floor. Bend one leg at approximately 100° and gradually pull the opposite leg toward your chest. Hold the final stretch for a few seconds. Switch legs and repeat the exercise.

Areas Stretched: Lower back and hamstring muscles, and lumbar spine ligaments.

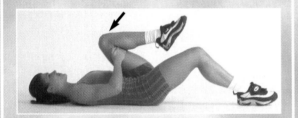

EXERCISE 32 — Double-Knee to Chest Stretch

Action: Lie flat on the floor and then slowly curl up into a fetal position. Hold for a few seconds.

Areas Stretched: Upper and lower back and hamstring muscles; spinal ligaments.

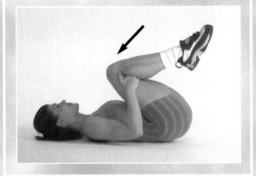

EXERCISE 33 — Upper and Lower Back Stretch

Action: Sit on the floor and bring your feet in close to you, allowing the soles of the feet to touch each other. Hold on to your feet and gently bring your head and upper chest toward your feet.

Areas Stretched: Upper and lower back muscles and ligaments.

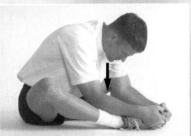

EXERCISE 34 — Sit-and-Reach Stretch

(see Exercise 29 in Appendix C)

EXERCISE 35 — Gluteal Stretch

Action: Sit on the floor, bend the left leg and place your left ankle slightly above the right knee. Grasp the right thigh with both hands and gently pull the leg toward your chest. Repeat the exercise with the opposite leg.

Areas Stretched: Buttock area (gluteal muscles).

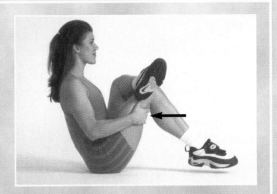

EXERCISE 36 — Back Extension

Action: Lie face down on the floor with the elbows by the chest, forearms on the floor, and the hands beneath the chin. Gently raise the trunk by extending the elbows until you reach an approximate 90° angle at the elbow joint. Be sure that the forearms remain in contact with the floor at all times. Hold the stretched position for a few seconds. DO NOT extend the back beyond this point. Hyperextension of the lower back may lead to or aggravate an already existing back problem.

Area Stretched: Abdominal region.

Additional Benefit: Restore lower back curvature.

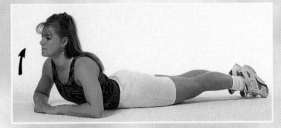

EXERCISE 37 — Trunk Rotation and Lower Back Stretch

Action: Sit on the floor and bend the right leg, placing the right foot on the outside of the left knee. Place the left elbow on the right knee and push against it. At the same time, try to rotate the trunk to the right (clockwise). Hold the final position for a few seconds. Repeat the exercise with the other side.

Areas Stretched: Lateral side of the hip and thigh; trunk, and lower back.

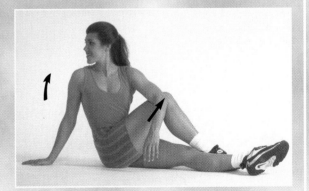

EXERCISE 38

Pelvic Tilt

Action: Lie flat on the floor with the knees bent at about a 90° angle. Tilt the pelvis by tightening the abdominal muscles, flattening your back against the floor, and raising the lower gluteal area ever so slightly off the floor (see illustration b). Hold the final position for several seconds. The exercise can also be performed against a wall (as shown in illustration c).

Areas Stretched: Low back muscles and ligaments.

Areas Strengthened: Abdominal and gluteal muscles.

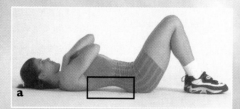

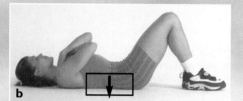

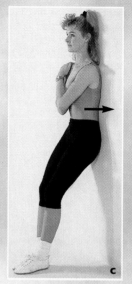

EXERCISE 39

The Cat

Action: Kneel on the floor and place your hands in front of you (on the floor) about shoulder width apart. Relax your trunk and lower back (a). Now arch the spine and pull in your abdomen as far as you can and hold this position for a few seconds (b). Repeat the exercise 4–5 times.

Areas Stretched: Low back muscles and ligaments.

Areas Strengthened: Abdominal and gluteal muscles.

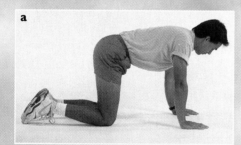

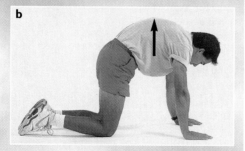

EXERCISE 40

Abdominal Crunch and Abdominal Curl-Up

(see Exercise 4 in Appendix B)

It is important that you do not stabilize your feet when performing either of these exercises, because doing so decreases the work of the abdominal muscles. Also, remember not to "swing up" but rather to curl up as you perform these exercises.

Caloric, Protein, Fat, Saturated Fat, Cholesterol, and Carbohydrate Content of Selected Foods*

Code	Food	Amount	Weight gm	Calories	Protein gm	Fat gm	Saturated Fat gm	Choles- terol mg	Carbohy- drate gm
1.	Almond Joy, candy bar	1.5 oz.	42	227	2.5	12	10.2	0	28
2.	Almonds, shelled	1/4 c	36	213	6.6	19	1.4	0	9
3.	Apple, raw, unpared	1 med	150	80	0.3	1	0.0	0	20
4.	Apple juice, canned or bottled	1/2 c	124	59	0.1	0	0.0	0	15
5.	Apple Pie, McDonald's	1	307	260	2	15	10.0	6	30
6.	Applesauce, canned, sweetened	1/2 c	128	116	0.3	0	0.0	0	31
7.	Apricots, canned, heavy syrup	3 halves; 1¾ tbsp liq.	85	73	0.5	0	0.0	0	19
8.	Apricots, dried, sulfured, uncooked	10 med halves	35	91	1.8	0	0.0	0	23
9.	Apricots, raw	3 (12 per lb)	114	55	1.1	0	0.0	0	14
10.	Arby Q, Arby's	1	190	389	18	15	5.5	29	48
11.	Arby Sauce, Arby's	.5 oz.	14	15	0	0	0.0	0	3
12.	Asparagus, cooked green spears	4 med	60	12	1.3	0	0.0	0	2
13.	Avocado, raw	1/2 med	120	185	2.4	19	3.2	0	7
14.	Bacon, cooked, drained	2 slices	15	86	3.8	8	2.7	30	1
15.	Bacon, lettuce, tomato sandwich	1	130	327	11.6	19	4.7	21	31
16.	Bagel	1 3½ in.	68	180	7.0	1	0.2	0	35
17.	Banana, raw	1 sm (7¼")	140	81	1.0	0	0.0	0	21
18.	Banana, nut bread	1 slice	50	169	3.0	8	1.5	33	22
19.	BBQ Sauce, McDonald's	1.12 oz.	32	50	0	0.6	0.2	0	12
20.	Beans, green snap, cooked	1/2 c	65	16	1.0	0	0.0	0	3
21.	Beans, lentils	1/4 c	50	53	3.9	0	0.0	0	10
22.	Beans, lima (Fordhook), froz., cooked	1/2 c	85	84	6.0	0	0.0	0	17
23.	Beans, red kidney, cooked	1 c	185	218	14.4	1	0.0	0	40
24.	Beans, refried	1/2 c	145	148	9.0	1	0.2	0	25
25.	Bean sprouts, mung, raw	1/2 c	52	18	2.0	0	0.0	0	4

From *Lifetime Physical Fitness & Wellness: A Personalized Program,* by Hoeger, W. W. K., Morton Publishing Company, 1995.

Code	Food	Amount	Weight gm	Calories	Protein gm	Fat gm	Saturated Fat gm	Choles- terol mg	Carbohy- drate gm
26.	Beef, chuck, cooked,	3 oz.	85	212	25.0	12	7.8	80	0
27.	Beef, corned, canned	3 oz.	85	163	21.0	10	8.0	70	0
28.	Beef, ground, lean	3 oz.	85	186	23.3	10	5.0	81	0
29.	Beef, Lite Roast Deluxe, Arby's	1	182	294	18	10	3.5	42	33
30.	Beef, meatloaf	1 piece	111	246	20.0	15	6.1	125	6
31.	Beef N' Cheddar, Arby's	1	194	508	25	27	7.7	52	43
32.	Beef, round steak, cooked, trimmed	3 oz.	85	222	24.3	13	6.0	77	0
33.	Beef, rump roast	3 oz.	85	177	24.7	9	4.0	80	0
34.	Beef, sirloin, cooked	3 oz.	85	329	19.6	27	13.0	77	0
35.	Beef, T-bone steak	3 oz.	85	403	16.7	37	15.6	66	0
36.	Beef, thin, sliced	3 oz.	85	105	18.5	3	1.4	36	0
37.	Beer	12 fl. oz.	360	151	1.1	0	1.1	0	14
38.	Beer, light	12 fl. oz.	354	96	0.7	0	0.0	0	4
39.	Beets, red, canned, drained	1/2 c	80	32	0.8	0	0.0	0	8
40.	Beet greens, cooked	1/2 c	73	13	1.3	0	0.0	0	2
41.	Biscuits, baking powder	1 med	35	114	2.5	6	1.1	0	18
42.	Blueberries, fresh cultivated	1/2 c	73	45	0.5	0	0.0	0	11
43.	Bologna	1 slice (1 oz.)	28	86	3.4	8	3.0	15	0
44.	Bologna, turkey	2 slices	57	113	7.8	9	3.0	56	1
45.	Bouillon, broth	1 cube	4	5	0.8	0	0.0	0	0
46.	Brandy	1 oz.	28	69	0.0	0	0.0	0	11
47.	Bread, Corn	1 slice	78	161	5.8	6	0.1	0	23
48.	Bread, Cracked wheat	1 slice	25	65	2.3	1	0.2	0	12
49.	Bread, French enriched	1 slice	35	102	3.2	1	0.2	0	19
50.	Bread, Oatmeal	1 slice	25	65	2.1	1	0.2	0	12
51.	Bread, Pita pocket	1 piece	60	165	6.2	1	0.1	0	33
52.	Bread, Pumpernickel	1 slice	32	80	2.9	1	0.2	0	15
53.	Bread, Rye (American)	1 slice	25	61	2.3	0	0.0	0	13
54.	Bread, white enriched	1 slice	25	68	2.2	1	0.2	0	13
55.	Bread, whole wheat	1 slice	25	61	2.6	1	0.6	0	12
56.	Broccoli, cooked drained	1 sm stalk	140	36	4.3	0	0.0	0	6
57.	Broccoli, raw	1 sm stalk	114	38	4.1	0	0.0	0	7
58.	Brownies, with nuts	1	20	95	1.3	6	2.3	18	11
59.	Brussels sprouts, froz., cooked, drained	1/2 c	78	28	3.2	0	0.0	0	5
60.	Bulgur, wheat	1 c	135	227	8.4	1	0.0	0	47
61.	Burrito, bean	1	166	307	12.5	9.5	3.6	14	45
62.	Burrito, combination, Taco Bell	1	175	404	21.0	16	0.0	0	43
63.	Butter	1 tsp	5	36	0.0	4	0.4	12	0
64.	Buttermilk, cultured	1 c	245	88	8.8	0	1.3	5	12
65.	Cabbage, boiled, drained wedge	1/2 c	85	16	0.9	0	0.0	0	3
66.	Cabbage, raw chopped	1/2 c	45	11	0.6	0	0.0	0	3
67.	Cake, Angel food, plain	1 piece	60	161	4.3	0	0.0	0	36
68.	Cake, Carrot	1 piece	96	385	4.2	21	4.1	74	48
69.	Cake, Cheesecake	1 piece (3½")	85	257	4.6	16	9.0	150	24
70.	Cake, Chocolate, w/icing	1 piece	69	235	3.0	8	3.6	37	40
71.	Cake, Coffee	1 piece	72	230	4.5	7	2.5	47	38
72.	Cake, Devil's food, iced	1 piece	99	365	4.5	16	5.0	68	55
73.	Cake, Pound	1 piece	30	120	2.0	5	1.0	32	15
74.	Cake, White, choc. icing	1 piece	71	268	3.5	11	3.7	2	48
75.	Candy, hard	1 oz.	28	109	0.0	0	0.0	0	28
76.	Cantaloupe	1/4 melon 5" diam.	239	35	2.0	0	0.0	0	10
77.	Caramel (candy, plain or choc.)	1 oz.	28	113	1.1	3	1.6	0	22
78.	Carrots, cooked, drained	1/2 c	73	23	0.7	0	0.0	0	5
79.	Carrots, raw	1 carrot 7½" long	81	30	0.8	0	0.0	0	7

Code	Food	Amount	Weight gm	Calories	Protein gm	Fat gm	Saturated Fat gm	Choles-terol mg	Carbohy-drate gm
80.	Cashew, roasted, unsalted	2 oz.	57	326	9.2	27	5.4	0	16
81.	Cauliflower, cooked, drained	1/2 c	63	14	1.5	0	0.0	0	3
82.	Celery, green, raw, long	1 outer stalk 8"	40	7	0.4	0	0.0	0	2
83.	Cereal, All-Bran	1/4 c	21	53	3.0	0	0.1	0	16
84.	Cereal, Alpha Bits	1 c	28	111	2.2	1	0.0	0	25
85.	Cereal, Bran	1/2 c	30	72	3.8	1	0.0	0	22
86.	Cereal, Cheerios	1 c	23	89	3.4	1	1.2	0	16
87.	Cereal, Corn Chex	1 c	28	111	2.0	0	0.1	0	25
88.	Cereal, Corn Flakes	1 c	25	97	2.0	0	0.0	0	21
89.	Cereal, Cream of Wheat	1 c	244	140	3.6	1	0.1	0	29
90.	Cereal, Frosted Mini-Wheats	4 biscuits	31	111	3.2	0	0.0	0	26
91.	Cereal, Fruit & Fibre w/dates	1 c	56	180	6.0	2	0.3	0	42
92.	Cereal, Granola, Nature Valley	1/2 c	57	252	5.8	10	7.0	0	38
93.	Cereal, Grape Nuts	1/2 c	57	202	6.6	0	0.0	0	47
94.	Cereal, Life	1 c	44	162	8.1	1	0.1	0	32
95.	Cereal, Nutri-Grain Wheat	1 c	44	158	3.8	1	0.1	0	37
96.	Cereal, Oatmeal, quick, cooked	1/2 c	120	66	2.4	1	0.2	0	12
97.	Cereal, Raisin Bran	1 c	49	160	4.0	1	0.2	0	40
98.	Cereal, Rice Krispies	3/4 c	22	85	1.4	0	0.0	0	19
99.	Cereal, Shredded Wheat	1 c	19	65	2.1	0	0.0	0	11
100.	Cereal, Special K	1 c	21	83	4.2	0	0.0	0	16
101.	Cereal, Sugar Corn Pops	1 c	28	108	1.4	0	0.0	0	26
102.	Cereal, Sugar Frosted Flakes	1 c	35	133	1.8	0	0.0	0	32
103.	Cereal, Sugar Smacks	1 c	37	141	2.7	1	0.1	0	32
104.	Cereal, Total	1 c	33	116	3.3	1	0.1	0	26
105.	Cereal, Wheat Chex	1 c	46	169	4.5	1	0.2	0	38
106.	Cereal, whole wheat, cooked	1/2 c	123	55	2.2	0	0.0	0	12
107.	Cereal, whole wheat flakes, ready-to-eat	1 c	30	106	3.1	1	0.0	0	24
108.	Cereal, 40% Bran Flakes	1 c	39	125	4.9	1	0.1	0	31
109.	Cereal, 100% Bran	1/2 c	33	89	4.2	2	0.3	0	24
110.	Champagne	4 oz.	113	87	0.2	0	0.1	0	2
111.	Cheese, American	1 oz. slice	28	100	6.0	8	5.6	27	0
112.	Cheese, Bleu	1 oz.	28	100	6.0	8	5.3	25	1
113.	Cheese, Cheddar	1 oz.	28	114	7.0	9	6.0	30	0
114.	Cheese, Cottage, 2%	1/2 c	113	103	15.5	2	1.4	10	4
115.	Cheese, Cottage, creamed	1/2 c	105	112	14.0	5	6.4	15	3
116.	Cheese, Creamed	1 oz.	28	99	6.0	8	3.0	31	1
117.	Cheese, Feta	1 oz.	28	75	4.5	6	4.2	25	1
118.	Cheese, Monterey jack	1 oz.	28	106	6.9	9	5.4	26	0
119.	Cheese, Mozzarella, skim	1 oz.	28	80	7.6	5	3.1	15	1
120.	Cheese, Parmesan	1 tbsp	5	23	2.1	2	1.0	4	0
121.	Cheese, Ricotta, part skim	1 oz.	28	39	3.2	2	1.4	9	1
122.	Cheese, Souffle	1 portion	110	240	10.9	19	9.5	189	7
123.	Cheese, Swiss	1 oz.	28	107	8.0	8	5.0	26	1
124.	Cheese puffs, Cheetos	1 oz.	28	158	2.2	10	4.8	5	14
125.	Cheeseburger, McDonald's	1	115	321	15.2	16	6.7	40	29
126.	Cherries	10	75	47	0.9	0	0.0	0	12
127.	Chicken, BK Broiler sandwich, Burger King	1 sandwich	168	379	24.0	18	3.0	53	31
128.	Chicken Breast Filet, Arby's	1	204	445	22	23.0	3.0	45	52
129.	Chicken breast, roast w/skin	1	98	193	29.2	8	2.1	83	0
130.	Chicken chow mein	1 c	250	255	31.0	11	3.6	75	10
131.	Chicken club sandwich, Wendy's	1	220	520	30	25	6.0	75	44
132.	Chicken Cordon Bleu, Arby's	1	225	518	30	27	5.3	92	52
133.	Chicken, drumstick Kentucky Fried	1	54	136	14.0	8	2.2	73	2

Code	Food	Amount	Weight gm	Calories	Protein gm	Fat gm	Saturated Fat gm	Choles-terol mg	Carbohy-drate gm
134.	Chicken, drumstick, roasted	1	52	112	14.1	6	1.6	48	0
135.	Chicken McNuggets	6	111	329	19.5	21	5.2	64	15
136.	Chicken Nuggets, Wendy's	6 pc.	94	280	14	20	5.0	50	12
137.	Chicken, patty sandwich	1	157	436	24.8	23	6.1	68	34
138.	Chicken, wing, Kentucky Fried	1	45	151	11.0	10	2.9	70	4
139.	Chicken, roast, light meat without skin	3 oz.	85	141	27.0	3	0.4	45	0
140.	Chicken, roast, dark meat without skin	3 oz.	85	149	24.0	5	0.8	50	0
141.	Chicken, Roast Deluxe, Arby's	1	195	276	24	7	1.7	33	33
142.	Chicken Sandwich, breaded Wendy's	1	208	450	26	20	4.0	60	44
143.	Chicken Sandwich, Grilled, Wendy's	1	177	290	24	7	1.0	60	35
144.	Chicken Sandwich, McChicken	1	187	415	19	19	9.0	50	39
145.	Chili con carne	1 c	255	339	19.1	16	5.8	28	31
146.	Chocolate fudge	1 oz.	28	115	0.6	3	2.1	1	21
147.	Chocolate, milk	1 oz.	28	147	2.0	9	3.6	5	16
148.	Chocolate, milk w/almonds	1 oz.	28	150	2.9	10	4.4	5	15
149.	Clam, canned, drained	3 oz.	85	83	13.0	2	0.2	50	2
150.	Cocoa, hot, with whole milk	1 c	250	218	9.1	9	6.1	33	26
151.	Cocoa, plain, dry	1 tbsp	5	14	0.9	1	0.0	0	3
152.	Coconut, shredded, packed	1/2 c	65	225	2.3	23	20.0	0	6
153.	Cod, batter fried	3.5 oz.	100	199	19.6	10	3.9	55	8
154.	Cod, cooked	3 oz.	85	144	24.3	4	1.5	60	0
155.	Cod, poached	3.5 oz.	100	94	20.9	1	0.3	60	0
156.	Coffee	3/4 cup	180	1	0.0	0	0.0	0	0
157.	Coleslaw	1 c	120	173	1.6	17	1.0	5	6
158.	Collards, leaves without stems, cooked, drained	1/2 c	95	32	3.4	1	2.0	0	5
159.	Cookies, Chocolate chip homemade	2 2¼" diam.	20	103	1.0	6	1.7	14	12
160.	Cookies, Fig bars	4 bars	56	210	2.0	4	1.0	27	42
161.	Cookies, Oatmeal raisin	2 2" diam.	26	122	1.5	5	1.3	1	18
162.	Cookies, Peanut butter, homemade	2 cookies	24	123	2.0	7	2.0	11	14
163.	Cookies, sandwich, all	4 cookies	40	195	2.0	8	2.0	0	29
164.	Cookies, Shortbread	4 cookies	32	155	2.0	8	2.9	27	20
165.	Cookies, Vanilla	5 1¾" diam.	20	93	1.0	3	0.8	10	15
166.	Cookies, Vanilla wafers	10 wafers	40	185	2.0	7	1.8	25	29
167.	Corn, boiled on cob	1 ear 5" long	140	70	2.5	1	0.0	0	16
168.	Corn, canned, drained	1/2 c	83	70	2.2	1	0.0	0	16
169.	Corn chips	1 oz.	28	155	2.0	9	1.8	0	16
170.	Cornmeal, degermed, yellow, enriched, cooked	1/2 c	120	60	1.3	0	0.0	0	13
171.	Crab, canned	1 c	135	135	23.0	3	0.5	135	1
172.	Crackers, Cheese	10 crackers	10	50	1.0	3	0.9	6	5
173.	Crackers, Graham	2 squares	14	55	1.1	1	0.3	0	10
174.	Crackers, Ritz	1 cracker	3	15	0.2	1	0.2	0	2
175.	Crackers, Ryewafers, whole grain	2 crackers	14	55	1.0	1	0.3	0	10
176.	Crackers, Saltines	4 squares	11	48	1.0	1	0.3	0	8
177.	Crackers, Soda	1	3	13	0.3	0	0.1	0	2
178.	Crackers, Triscuits	1	5	23	0.4	1	0.3	0	3
179.	Crackers, Wheat Thins	1	2	9	0.2	0	0.1	0	1
180.	Cranberry juice	1 c	253	145	0.1	0	0.0	0	36
181.	Cream, light coffee or table	1 tbsp	15	20	0.5	2	0.5	5	1
182.	Cream, heavy whipping	1 tbsp	15	53	0.3	6	1.3	12	1

Code	Food	Amount	Weight gm	Calories	Protein gm	Fat gm	Saturated Fat gm	Cholesterol mg	Carbohydrate gm
183.	Croissant	1	57	235	4.7	12	4.0	13	27
184.	Croissants (Sara Lee)	1 roll	18	59	1.6	2	0.3	0	8
185.	Croissan'wich, egg, cheese Burger King	1 sandwich	110	315	13.0	20	7.0	222	19
186.	Cucumbers, raw pared	9 sm slices	28	4	0.3	0	0.0	0	1
187.	Danish, Apple, McDonald's	1	115	390	6	17	11.0	25	51
188.	Danish, Cinnamon Raisin	1	110	440	6	21	13.0	34	58
189.	Dates hydrated	5	46	110	0.9	0	0.0	0	29
190.	Doughnut, plain	1	42	164	1.9	8	2.0	19	22
191.	Doughnut, yeast raised	1	27	235	4.0	13	5.2	21	26
192.	Dressing, Bleu cheese	1 tbsp	15	77	0.7	8	1.9	4	1
193.	Dressing, French	1 tbsp	16	83	0.1	9	1.4	0	1
194.	Dressing, French, low cal	1 tbsp.	15	24	0.0	2	0.2	0	2
195.	Dressing, Italian	1 tbsp.	15	69	0.1	9	1.3	0	2
196.	Dressing, Italian, low cal	1 tbsp.	15	10	0.0	1	0.0	0	1
197.	Dressing, Ranch style	1 tbsp.	15	54	0.4	6	0.9	6	1
198.	Dressing, Thousand island	1 tbsp.	15	60	0.2	6	1.0	4	2
199.	Dressing, Thousand island, low cal	1 tbsp.	15	25	0.1	2	0.2	2	3
200.	Egg, hard cooked	1 large	50	72	6.0	5	1.6	212	1
201.	Egg, fried with butter	1	46	95	5.4	7	2.4	240	1
202.	Egg McMuffin	1	138	327	18.5	15	5.9	259	31
203.	Egg salad sandwich	1	111	325	10.0	19	3.9	215	28
204.	Egg, scrambled, with milk, butter	1 egg	64	95	6.0	7	3.0	244	1
205.	Egg, white	1 large	33	17	3.6	0	0.0	0	0
206.	Egg, yolk, raw	1 yolk	17	63	2.8	5	1.6	212	0
207.	Enchilada, beef	1	200	487	21.8	23	8.8	63	26
208.	Enchilada, cheese	1	230	632	25.3	34	17.6	82	31
209.	Figs, dried	1 large	21	60	1.0	0	0.0	0	15
210.	Filet of Fish, McDonald's	1	131	402	15.0	23	7.9	43	34
211.	Fish sandwich, Wendy's	1	182	460	16	25	5.0	55	42
212.	Fish, sticks	2	56	140	12.0	6	1.6	52	8
213.	Flounder	3 oz.	85	171	25.5	7	1.0	60	0
214.	Flour, all purpose enriched	1 c	125	455	13.0	1	0.0	0	95
215.	Flour, whole wheat	1 c	120	400	16.0	2	0.0	0	85
216.	Frankfurter, cooked	1	57	176	7.0	16	5.6	45	1
217.	Frankfurter, turkey, cooked	1	45	102	6.4	8	2.7	39	1
218.	French Dip, Arby's	1	154	368	22	15	5.6	43	35
219.	French toast	1 piece	65	123	4.9	4	1.1	73	15
220.	Fries, Curly, Arby's	1 small	99	337	4	18	7.4	0	43
221.	Fruit cocktail	1 c	245	91	1.0	0	0.0	0	24
222.	Fruit cocktail, juice pack	1 c	248	115	1.1	0	0.0	0	29
223.	Grapefruit, raw white	1/2 med	301	56	1.0	0	0.0	0	15
224.	Grapefruit juice, unsweet. canned	1/2 c	124	50	0.6	0	0.0	0	12
225.	Grapes, seedless, European	10 grapes	50	34	0.3	0	0.0	0	9
226.	Grape juice, unsweetened bottled	1/2 c	127	84	0.3	0	0.0	0	21
227.	Gravy, beef, homemade	1 tbsp	17	19	0.3	2	1.0	1	1
228.	Haddock, fried (dipped in egg, milk, bread crumbs)	3 oz.	85	141	17.0	5	1.0	54	5
229.	Halibut, broiled with butter or margarine	3 oz.	85	144	21.0	6	2.1	55	0
230.	Ham (cured pork)	3 oz.	85	318	20.0	26	9.4	77	0
231.	Ham, lunch meat	1 slice	28	37	5.5	1	0.5	13	.3
232.	Hamburger, Big Classic, Wendy's	1	251	480	27	23	7.0	75	44
233.	Hamburger, Big Mac	1	204	581	25.1	36	12.0	85	40
234.	Hamburger bun	1 bun	40	129	3.7	2	1.0	0	23
235.	Hamburger, Jr. Bacon Cheeseburger, Wendy's	1	170	440	22	25	8.0	65	33
236.	Hamburger, McDonald's	1	99	257	13.0	9	3.7	26	30

Code	Food	Amount	Weight gm	Calories	Protein gm	Fat gm	Saturated Fat gm	Cholesterol mg	Carbohydrate gm
237.	Hamburger, McLean Deluxe	1	206	320	22	10	5.0	60	35
238.	Hamburger, McLean Deluxe, w/cheese	1	219	370	24	14	8.0	75	35
239.	Hamburger, Quarter pounder	1 burger	160	427	24.6	24	9.1	80	29
240.	Hamburger, Quarter pounder, with cheese	1 burger	186	525	29.6	32	12.8	107	31
241.	Hamburger, Wendy's	1	219	440	26	23	7.0	75	36
242.	Ham N' Cheese, Arby's	1	169	355	25	14	5.1	55	35
243.	Honey	1 tbsp	21	64	0.0	0	0.0	0	17
244.	Honeydew melon	1 slice (1/10 melon)	129	45	0.6	0	0.0	0	12
245.	Horsey Sauce, Arby's	.5 oz.	14	55	0	5	2.0	0	3
246.	Hotcakes w/Margarine & Syrup, McDonald's	1 serving	174	440	8	12	5.0	8	74
247.	Hotdog bun	1 bun	40	115	3.3	2	1.0	0	20
248.	Ice cream, vanilla	1/2 c	67	135	3.0	7	4.4	27	14
249.	Ice cream cone	1 small	115	185	4.3	5	2.2	24	30
250.	Ice cream cone, Dairy Queen	medium	142	230	6.0	7	4.6	15	35
251.	Ice cream, hot fudge sundae	1	164	357	7.0	11	5.4	27	58
252.	Ice milk, vanilla	1/2 c	61	100	3.0	3	1.8	13	15
253.	Instant breakfast, whole milk	1 c	281	280	15.0	8	5.1	33	34
254.	Instant breakfast, skim milk	1 c	282	216	15.4	0	0.0	4	35
255.	Jams or preserves	1 tbsp	7	18	0.0	0	0.0	0	5
256.	Jelly	1 tbsp	18	49	0.0	0	0.0	0	13
257.	Kale, fresh cooked, drained	1/2 c	55	22	2.5	0	0.0	0	3
258.	Kiwi fruit, raw	1 med	76	46	1.0	0	0.0	0	11
259.	Kool Aid, with sugar	1 c	240	100	0.0	0	0.0	0	25
260.	Lamb leg, roast, trimmed	3 oz.	85	237	22.0	16	7.3	60	0
261.	Lamb loin chop, broiled, lean	3 oz.	84	183	25.0	8	3.4	78	0
262.	Lasagna, homemade	1 piece	220	357	23.6	18	8.3	50	27
263.	Lemon juice, fresh	1 tbsp	15	4	0.1	0	0.0	0	1
264.	Lemonade (concentrate)	12 oz.	340	137	0.2	0	0.1	0	36
265.	Lentils, cooked	1/2 c	100	106	8.0	0	0.0	0	19
266.	Lettuce, crisp head	1 c sm chunks	75	10	0.7	0	0.0	0	2
267.	Lettuce, cos or romaine	1 c chopped	55	10	0.7	0	0.0	0	2
268.	Liver, beef, fried	1 slice 3 oz.	85	195	22.0	9	2.5	345	5
269.	Liverwurst, fresh	1 slice 1 oz.	28	87	5.0	7	3.5	50	1
270.	Lobster	1 c	145	138	27.0	2	1.0	293	0
271.	M&M's, Chocolate, plain	1 oz.	28	140	1.9	6	3.3	0	19
272.	M&M's, Chocolate, w/peanuts	1 oz.	28	145	3.2	7	3.2	0	17
273.	Macaroni, enriched, cooked	1/2 c	70	78	2.4	0	0.0	0	16
274.	Macaroni and cheese	1/2 c	100	215	8.2	11	4.0	21	20
275.	Margarine	1 tsp	5	34	0.0	4	0.7	2	0
276.	Mars bar	1 bar	50	240	4.0	11	4.8	0	30
277.	Matzo	1 piece	30	117	3.0	0	0.0	0	25
278.	Mayonnaise	1 tsp	5	36	0.0	4	0.7	3	0
279.	Milk, chocolate, 2%	1 c	250	180	8.0	5	3.1	17	26
280.	Milk, evaporated whole	1/2 c	126	172	9.0	10	5.8	40	13
281.	Milk, lowfat 2% fat	1 c	246	145	10	5	3.1	5	15
282.	Milk shake, chocolate	1 (10 fluid oz.)	340	433	11.5	13	7.8	45	70
283.	Milk shake, Frosty, Wendy's	16 oz.	324	460	13	13	7.0	55	76
284.	Milk shake, strawberry	1 (10 fluid oz.)	340	383	11.4	10	6.0	37	64
285.	Milk shake, vanilla, McDonald's	1	289	323	10	8	5.1	29	52
286.	Milk, skim	1 c	245	88	9.0	0	0.3	5	12
287.	Milk, whole 3.5% fat	1 c	244	159	9.0	9	5.1	34	12
288.	Milky Way bar	1 bar	60	260	3.2	9	5.4	14	43
289.	Molasses, medium	1 tbsp	20	50	0.0	0	0.0	0	13
290.	Muffin, apple bran, fat free, McDonald's	1	75	180	5	0	0.0	0	40

Code	Food	Amount	Weight gm	Calories	Protein gm	Fat gm	Saturated Fat gm	Choles-terol mg	Carbohy-drate gm
291.	Muffin, blueberry	1	45	135	3.0	5	1.5	19	20
292.	Muffin, bran	1	45	125	3.0	6	1.4	24	19
293.	Muffin, cornmeal	1	45	145	3.0	5	1.5	23	21
294.	Muffin, English, plain	1	57	140	4.5	1	0.3	0	26
295.	Muffin, English w/butter	1	63	186	5.0	5	2.3	15	30
296.	Mushrooms, fresh cultivated	1/2 c sliced	35	12	1.0	0	0.0	0	2
297.	Mustard greens, cooked drained	1/2 c	70	16	1.7	0	0.0	0	3
298.	Noodles, egg, enriched cooked	1/2 c	80	100	3.3	1	0.0	0	19
299.	Nuts, Brazil	1 oz. (6-8 nuts)	28	185	4.1	19	4.8	0	3
300.	Nuts, Pecans	1 oz.	28	195	2.6	20	1.4	0	4
301.	Nuts, Walnuts	1 oz. (14 halves)	28	185	4.2	18	1.0	0	5
302.	Oil, Corn	1 tbsp.	15	125	0.0	14	1.8	0	0
303.	Oil, Olive	1 tbsp.	15	125	0.0	14	1.9	0	0
304.	Oil, Safflower	1 tbsp.	15	125	0.0	14	1.3	0	0
305.	Oil, Soybean	1 tsp.	5	44	0.0	5	2.0	0	0
306.	Okra, cooked, drained	1/2 c	80	23	1.6	0	0.0	0	5
307.	Olives, black, ripe	10 extra large	55	61	0.5	7	1.0	0	1
308.	Onions, mature,	1/2 c sliced	105	31	1.3	0	0.0	0	7
309.	cooked, drained								
310.	Onion rings, fried	3	30	122	1.6	8	2.3	0	11
311.	Onion rings (Brazier) Dairy Queen	1 serving	85	360	6.0	17	6.0	15	33
312.	Orange juice, froz. reconstituted	1/2 c	125	61	0.9	0	0.0	0	15
313.	Orange, raw (medium skin)	1 med	180	64	1.3	0	0.0	0	16
314.	Oysters, Eastern, breaded, fried	1 oyster	45	90	5.0	5	1.4	35	5
315.	Oysters, raw, Eastern	1/2 c (6-9 med)	120	79	10.0	2	1.3	60	4
316.	Pancakes	1 6" diam x 1/2" thick	73	169	5.2	5	1.0	36	25
317.	Pancakes, buckwheat	1 4 in. diam.	27	55	2.0	2	0.9	20	6
318.	Pancakes w/butter, syrup	1 large	100	250	4.0	5	1.9	24	47
319.	Papaya, raw	1/2 med	227	60	0.9	0	0.0	0	15
320.	Parsnips, cooked	1 large 9" long	160	106	2.4	1	0.0	0	24
321.	Peaches, canned, heavy syrup	1 half 2⅛ tbsp liq.	96	75	0.4	0	0.0	0	19
322.	Peaches, canned, juice pack	1 half	77	34	0.5	0	0.0	0	9
323.	Peaches, raw, peeled	1 2¾" diam.	175	58	0.9	0	0.0	0	15
324.	Peanut butter	2 tbsp	32	188	8.0	16	1.0	0	6
325.	Peanut butter, jam sandwich	1	100	340	11.4	14	2.6	0	45
326.	Peanuts, roasted	1 oz.	28	166	7.0	14	1.0	0	5
327.	Pears, canned, heavy syrup	1 half 2¼ tbsp liq.	103	78	0.2	0	0.0	0	20
328.	Pears, canned, juice pack	1 half	77	38	0.3	0	0.0	0	10
329.	Pears, raw	1 pear	180	100	1.1	1	0.0	0	25
330.	Peas, canned, drained	1/2 c	85	75	4.0	0	0.0	0	14
331.	Peas, frozen, cooked drained	1/2 c	80	55	4.1	0	0.0	0	10
332.	Peppers, sweet, raw	1 pepper 3¼" x 3" diam.	200	36	2.0	0	0.0	0	8
333.	Pickles, dill	1 large 4" long	135	15	0.9	0	0.0	0	3
334.	Pickles, sweet	1 large 3" long	35	51	0.2	0	0.0	0	13
335.	Pie, Apple	1 piece (3½")	118	302	2.6	13	3.5	120	45
336.	Pie, Apple, fried	1 pie	85	255	2.2	14	5.8	14	32
337.	Pie, Blueberry	1 piece (3½")	158	380	4.0	17	4.0	0	55
338.	Pie, Cherry	1 piece (3½")	118	308	3.1	13	5.0	137	45
339.	Pie, Cherry, fried	1 pie	85	250	2.0	14	5.8	13	32
340.	Pie, Chocolate cream	1 piece (1/6 pie)	175	311	7.4	13	4.5	15	42
341.	Pie, Lemon meringue	1 piece (1/6 pie)	140	355	4.7	14	3.5	137	53
342.	Pie, Pecan	1 piece (1/6 pie)	138	583	6.3	24	3.9	13	92

Code	Food	Amount	Weight gm	Calories	Protein gm	Fat gm	Saturated Fat gm	Cholesterol mg	Carbohydrate gm
343.	Pie, Pumpkin	1 (3½")	114	241	4.6	13	3.0	70	28
344.	Pineapple, canned, heavy syrup	1/2 c	128	95	0.4	0	0.0	0	25
345.	Pineapple, canned, juice pack	1/2 c	125	75	0.5	0	0.0	0	20
346.	Pineapple, raw	1/2 c diced	78	41	0.3	0	0.0	0	11
347.	Pizza, Cheese, Thin 'n Crispy, Pizza Hut	1/2 10" pie	*	450	25.0	15	7.0	125	54
348.	Pizza, Cheese, Thick 'n Chewy, Pizza Hut	1/2 10" pie	*	560	34.0	14	6.0	110	71
349.	Plums, Japanese and hybrid, raw	1 plum 2⅛" diam.	70	32	0.3	0	0.0	0	8
350.	Popcorn, cooked, oil	1 c	11	55	0.9	3	0.5	0	6
351.	Popcorn, popped, plain, large kernel	1 c	6	12	0.8	0	0.0	0	5
352.	Pork, roast, trimmed	2 slices 3 oz.	85	179	24.0	8	2.2	65	0
353.	Pork, sausage, cooked	1 sm link	17	72	2.8	6	2.1	13	1
354.	Potato, au gratin	1 c	245	228	5.6	10	6.3	12	32
355.	Potato, baked in skin	1 potato 2⅓ x 4¼"	202	145	4.0	0	0.0	0	33
356.	Potato chips	10 chips	20	114	1.1	8	2.1	0	10
357.	Potato, French fried long	10 strips 3½-4"	78	214	3.4	10	1.7	0	28
358.	Potato, Hashbrowns, McDonald's	1 patty	55	144	1.4	9	3.0	4	15
359.	Potato, mashed, milk added	1/2 c	105	69	2.2	1	0.4	8	14
360.	Potato salad w/eggs, mayo	1/2 c	125	179	3.4	10	7.8	85	14
361.	Potato, hash brown	1/2 c	78	170	2.5	9	3.5	0	22
362.	Pretzel, thin, twists	1 oz.	28	113	2.8	1	0.3	0	23
363.	Prunes, dried "softenized" without pits	5 prunes	61	137	1.1	0	0.0	0	36
364.	Prune juice, canned or bottled	1/2 c	128	99	0.5	0	0.0	0	24
365.	Pudding, Chocolate, canned	5 oz.	142	205	3	11	9.5	1	30
366.	Pudding, Tapioca, canned	5 oz.	142	160	3	5	4.8	1	28
367.	Pudding, Vanilla, canned	5 oz.	142	220	2	10	9.5	1	33
368.	Quiche, Lorraine	1 piece	242	825	18	66	31.9	392	40
369.	Raisins, unbleached, seedless	1 oz.	28	82	0.7	0	0.0	0	22
370.	Raspberries, fresh	1 c	123	60	1.1	1	0.0	0	14
371.	Raspberries, frozen	1 c	250	255	1.7	1	0.0	0	62
372.	Rice, brown, cooked	1/2 c	96	116	2.5	1	0.0	0	25
373.	Rice, white enriched, cooked	1/2 c	103	113	2.1	0	0.0	0	25
374.	Rice, wild, cooked	1/2 c	100	92	3.6	0	0.0	0	19
375.	Roast Beef sand., Regular, Arby's	1	155	383	22	18	7.0	43	35
376.	Roast Beef Sub, Arby's	1	305	623	38	32	11.5	73	47
377.	Roll, hard, white	1 roll	50	155	5	2	0.0	0	30
378.	Reuben sandwich	1	237	488	28.7	28	10.4	85	30
379.	Salad, Caesar side, Wendy's	1	130	160	10	6	1.0	10	18
380.	Salad, Chef, Burger King	1 serving	273	178	17	9	4.0	103	7
381.	Salad, Chef, McDonald's	1	265	170	17	9	4.0	111	8
382.	Salad, Chicken, Burger King	1 serving	258	142	20	4	1.0	49	8
383.	Salad, Chicken w/celery	1/2 c	78	266	10.5	25	4.1	48	1
384.	Salad, Deluxe Garden, Wendy's	1	271	110	7	5	1.0	0	9
385.	Salad, Garden, Arby's	1	330	117	7	5	2.7	12	11
386.	Salad, Grilled Chicken, Wendy's	1	338	200	25	8	1.0	55	9
387.	Salad, Tuna	1 c	205	375	33	19	3.3	80	19
388.	Salami, dry	1 oz.	28	128	7.0	11	1.6	24	0
389.	Salmon, broiled with butter or margarine	3 oz.	85	156	23.0	6	2.2	53	0
390.	Salmon, canned Chinook	3 oz.	85	179	16.6	12	0.8	30	0
391.	Sardines, canned drained	1 oz.	28	58	7.0	3	1.0	20	0
392.	Sauerkraut, canned	1/2 c	118	21	1.2	0	0.0	0	5
393.	Sausage Biscuit w/Egg, McDonald's	1	175	505	19	33	20.0	260	33

Code	Food	Amount	Weight gm	Calories	Protein gm	Fat gm	Saturated Fat gm	Cholesterol mg	Carbohydrate gm
394.	Sausage McMuffin, McDonald's	1	135	345	15	20	11.0	57	27
395.	Sausage McMuffin, w/Egg	1	159	430	21	25	14.0	270	27
396.	Sausage, smoked link, pork	1	68	265	15	22	7.7	46	1
397.	Scallops, breaded, cooked	6 pieces	90	195	15	10	2.5	70	10
398.	Sherbet	1/2 c	97	135	1.1	2	1.3	7	29
399.	Shrimp, boiled	3 oz.	85	99	18.0	1	0.1	128	1
400.	Shrimp, fried	7 medium	85	200	16.0	10	2.5	168	11
401.	Snickers bar	1 bar	61	290	6.6	4	5.4	0	37
402.	Soda pop, cola	12 oz.	369	144	0.0	0	0.0	0	37
403.	Soda pop, diet	12 oz.	340	2	0.1	0	0.0	0	0
404.	Soda pop, Ginger ale	12 oz.	366	113	0.0	0	0.0	0	29
405.	Soda pop, Lemon-lime	12 oz.	340	138	0.0	0	0.0	0	35
406.	Soda pop, Root beer	12 oz.	340	140	0.0	0	0.0	0	36
407.	Soup, Chicken, cream	1 c	248	191	7.5	12	4.6	27	15
408.	Soup, Chicken noodle	1 c	241	75	4.0	2	0.7	7	9
409.	Soup, Clam chowder, Manhattan	1 c	244	78	4.2	2	0.4	2	12
410.	Soup, Clam chowder, north east	1 c	248	163	9.5	7	3.0	22	16
411.	Soup, Cream of mushroom condensed, prepared with equal volume of milk	1 c	245	216	7.0	14	5.4	15	16
412.	Soup, Minestrone	1 c	241	80	4.3	3	0.5	2	11
413.	Soup, Split pea, condensed, prepared with equal volume of water	1 c	245	145	9.0	3	1.1	0	21
414.	Soup, Tomato, condensed, prepared with equal volume of water	1 c	245	88	2.0	3	0.5	0	16
415.	Soup, Tomato with milk	1 c	248	160	6.0	6	2.9	17	22
416.	Soup, vegetable beef, condensed, prepared with equal volume of water	1 c	245	78	5.0	2	0.0	0	10
417.	Soup, Vegetarian vegetable	1 c	250	70	2.1	2	0.3	0	12
418.	Sour cream	1 tbsp	14	30	0.4	3	1.8	6	1
419.	Soup cream, imitation	1 tbsp.	14	29	0.3	3	2.5	0	1
420.	Spaghetti, in tomato sauce with cheese	1 c	250	260	8.8	9	2.0	10	37
421.	Spaghetti, plain, cooked	1 c	140	155	5.0	1	0.1	0	32
422.	Spaghetti, whole wheat, cooked	1 c	125	151	6.6	1	0.1	0	32
423.	Spaghetti, with meatballs and tomato sauce	1 c	248	332	18.6	11.7	3.0	75	39
424.	Spareribs, cooked	3 oz.	85	377	17.8	33	12.0	73	0
425.	Spinach, canned, drained	1/2 c	103	25	2.3	1	0.0	0	4
426.	Spinach, frozen, cooked, drained	1/2 c	103	24	3.1	0	0.0	0	4
427.	Spinach, raw, chopped	1 c	55	14	1.8	0	0.0	0	2
428.	Squash, summer, cooked	1/2 c	90	13	0.8	0	0.0	0	3
429.	Squash, winter, baked mashed	1/2 c	103	70	1.9	0	0.0	0	18
430.	Strawberries, frozen, sweetened	1 c	250	245	1.4	0	0.0	0	66
431.	Strawberries, raw	1 c	149	55	1.0	1	0.0	0	13
432.	Stuffing, bread, prepared	1/2 c	70	250	4.6	15	3.1	0	25
433.	Sundae, choc. Dairy Queen	medium	184	300	6.0	7	4.9	79	53
434.	Sugar, brown granulated	1 tsp	5	17	0.0	0	0.0	0	5
435.	Sugar, white granulated	1 tsp	4	15	0.0	0	0.0	0	4
436.	Super Roast Beef, Arby's	1	254	552	24	28	7.6	43	54
437.	Sweet N' Sour Sauce, McDonalds	1.12 oz.	32	60	0	0.2	0.1	0	14
438.	Sweet potato, baked	1 potato 5" long	146	161	2.4	1	0.0	0	37
439.	Syrup (maple)	1 tbsp	20	50	0.0	0	0.0	0	13
440.	Taco Salad, Wendy's	1	510	640	34	30	12.0	80	70

Code	Food	Amount	Weight gm	Calories	Protein gm	Fat gm	Saturated Fat gm	Choles- terol mg	Carbohy- drate gm
441.	Taco shell	1 shell	10	60	1.1	3	0.3	0	9
442.	Taco, Taco Bell	1	83	186	15.0	8	0.0	0	14
443.	Tangerine	1 med 2⅛" diam.	116	39	0.7	0	0.0	0	10
444.	Tartar sauce	1 tbsp.	14	74	0.2	8	1.2	4	1
445.	Tea, brewed	1/4 c	180	0	0.0	0	0.0	0	0
446.	Tomato juice, canned	1 c	244	42	1.9	0	0.1	0	10
447.	Tomato sauce (catsup)	1 tbsp	15	16	0.3	0	0.0	0	4
448.	Tomato, canned	1/2 c	121	26	1.2	0	0.0	0	5
449.	Tomato, raw	1 tomato 3½ oz.	100	20	1.0	0	0.0	0	4
450.	Tortilla chips	1 oz.	28	139	2.2	8	1.1	0	17
451.	Tortilla, corn, lime	1 6" diam.	30	63	1.5	1	0.0	0	14
452.	Tortilla, flour	1	35	105	2.6	3	0.4	0	19
453.	Tostada	1	148	206	9.2	18	3.0	14	25
454.	Trout, broiled w/butter, lemon	3 oz.	85	175	21.0	9	4.1	71	0
455.	Tuna, canned, oil pack, drained	3 oz.	85	167	25.0	7	1.7	60	0
456.	Tuna, canned, water pack, solids and liquid	3½ oz.	99	126	27.7	1	0.0	55	0
457.	Turkey, Lite Roast Deluxe, Arby's	1	195	260	20	6	1.6	33	33
458.	Turkey, roast (light and dark mixed)	3 oz.	85	162	27.0	5	1.5	73	0
459.	Turnip, cooked, drained	1/2 c cubed	78	18	0.6	0	0.0	0	4
460.	Turnip greens, cooked drained	1/2 c	73	19	2.1	0	0.0	0	3
461.	Veal, cooked loin	3 oz.	85	199	22.0	11	4.0	90	0
462.	Veal cutlet, braised, broiled	3 oz.	85	185	23.0	9	4.0	109	0
463.	Vegetables, mixed, cooked	1 c	182	116	5.8	0	0.0	0	24
464.	Waffles	1 waffle	75	205	6.9	8	2.7	59	27
465.	Watermelon	1 c diced	160	42	0.8	0	0.0	0	10
466.	Wheat germ, plain toasted	1 tbsp	6	23	1.8	1	0.0	0	3
467.	Whiskey, gin, rum, vodka 90 proof	1/2 11 oz (jigger)	42	110	0	0	0.0	0	0
468.	Whopper, Burger King	1 sandwich	270	614	27.0	36	12.0	90	45
469.	Whopper with cheese, Burger King	1 sandwich	294	706	32.0	44	16.0	115	47
470.	Whopper, double, Burger King	1 sandwich	351	844	46.0	53	19.0	169	45
471.	Wine, dry table 12% alc.	3½ fl. oz.	102	87	0.1	0	0.0	0	4
472.	Wine, red dry 18.8% alc.	2 oz.	59	81	0.1	0	0.0	0	5
473.	Yeast, brewers	1 tbsp	8	23	3.1	0	0.0	0	3
474.	Yogurt, fruit	1 c	227	231	9.9	2	1.6	10	43
475.	Yogurt, nonfat, TCBY	4 oz.	113	110	4	0	0	0	23
476.	Yogurt, plain low fat	1 8-oz. container	226	113	7.7	4	2.3	15	12
477.	Yogurt, regular, TCBY	4 oz.	113	120	4	3	2.0	13	23
478.	Yogurt, sugar free, TCBY	4 oz.	113	80	4	0	0	0	18
479.	Yogurt, vanilla lowfat, McDonald's	3 oz.	85	105	4	1	0.3	3	22

"0" represents both less than 1 and 0

Sources:

Nutritive Value of American Foods in Common Units. *Agriculture Handbook No. 456*. U.S. Dept. of Agriculture. Washington, D.C. 1988.

Young, E. A., E. H. Brennan, and C. L. Irving, Guest Eds. Perspectives on Fast Foods. *Public Health Currents*, 19(1), 1979, Published by Ross Laboratories, Columbus, OH.

Dennison, D. *The Dine System: the Nutrition Plan For Better Health*. C. V. Mosby Company St. Louis, Missouri, 1982.

Pennington, S. A. T. and H. N. Church. *Food Values of Portions Commonly Used*. Harper and Row Publishers, New York, 1985.

Kullman, D. A. *ABC Milligram Cholesterol Diet Guide*. Merit Publications, Inc. North Miami Beach, Florida 1978.

Food Processor nutrient analysis software by Esha Corporation, P.O. Box 13028, Salem, Oregon, 97309. With permission.

Healthstyle: A Self-Test

All of us want good health. But many of us do not know how to be as healthy as possible. Health experts now describe *lifestyle* as one of the most important factors affecting health. In fact, it is estimated that as many as seven of the ten leading causes of death could be reduced through common-sense changes in lifestyle. That's what this brief test, developed by the Public Health Service, is all about. Its purpose is simply to tell you how well you are doing to stay healthy. The behaviors covered in the test are recommended for most Americans. Some of them may not apply to persons with certain chronic diseases or handicaps, or to pregnant women. Such persons may require special instructions from their physicians.

Cigarette Smoking

If you *never smoke*, enter a score of 10 for this section and go to the next section on *Alcohol and Drugs*.

	Almost Always	Sometimes	Almost Never
1. I avoid smoking cigarettes.	2	1	0
2. I smoke only low tar and nicotine cigarettes *or* I smoke a pipe or cigars.	2	1	0

Smoking Score: _10_

Source: National Health Information Clearinghouse. Washington, D.C.

Alcohol and Drugs

	Almost Always	Sometimes	Almost Never
1. I avoid drinking alcoholic beverages *or* I drink no more than 1 or 2 drinks a day.	4	1	0
2. I avoid using alcohol or other drugs (especially illegal drugs) as a way of handling stressful situations or the problems in my life.	2	1	0
3. I am careful not to drink alcohol when taking certain medicines (for example, medicine for sleeping, pain, colds, and allergies), or when pregnant.	2	1	0
4. I read and follow the label directions when using prescribed and over-the-counter drugs.	2	1	0

Alcohol and Drugs Score: 10

Eating Habits

	Almost Always	Sometimes	Almost Never
1. I eat a variety of foods each day, such as fruits and vegetables, whole grain breads and cereals, lean meats, dairy products, dry peas and beans, and nuts and seeds.	4	1	0
2. I limit the amount of fat, saturated fat, and cholesterol I eat (including fat on meats, eggs, butter, cream, shortenings, and organ meats such as liver).	2	1	0
3. I limit the amount of salt I eat by cooking with only small amounts, not adding salt at the table, and avoiding salty snacks.	2	1	0
4. I avoid eating too much sugar (especially frequent snacks of sticky candy or soft drinks).	2	1	0

Eating Habits Score: 10

Exercise/Fitness

		Almost Always	Sometimes	Almost Never
1.	I maintain a desired weight, avoiding overweight and underweight.	3	1	0
2.	I do vigorous exercises for 20–30 minutes at least 3 times a week (examples include running, swimming, brisk walking).	3	1	0
3.	I do exercises that enhance my muscle tone for 15–30 minutes at least 3 times a week (examples include yoga and calisthenics).	2	1	0
4.	I use part of my leisure time participating in individual, family, or team activities that increase my level of fitness (such as gardening, bowling, golf, and baseball).	2	1	0

Exercise/Fitness Score: _____2_____

Stress Control

		Almost Always	Sometimes	Almost Never
1.	I have a job or do other work that I enjoy.	2	1	0
2.	I find it easy to relax and express my feelings freely.	2	1	0
3.	I recognize early, and prepare for, events or situations likely to be stressful for me.	2	1	0
4.	I have close friends, relatives, or others whom I can talk to about personal matters and call on for help when needed.	2	1	0
5.	I participate in group activities (such as church and community organizations) or hobbies that I enjoy.	2	1	0

Stress Control Score: _____8_____

Safety

	Almost Always	Sometimes	Almost Never
1. I wear a seat belt while riding in a car.	2	1	0
2. I avoid driving while under the influence of alcohol and other drugs.	2	1	0
3. I obey traffic rules and the speed limit when driving.	2	1	0
4. I am careful when using potentially harmful products or substances (such as household cleaners, poisons, and electrical devices).	2	1	0
5. I avoid smoking in bed.	2	1	0

Safety Score: 10 _____

What Your Scores Mean to YOU

Scores of 9 and 10   Excellent! Your answers show that you are aware of the importance of this area to your health. More important, you are putting your knowledge to work for you by practicing good health habits. As long as you continue to do so, this area should not pose a serious health risk. It's likely that you are setting an example for your family and friends to follow. Since you got a very high test score on this part of the test, you may want to consider other areas where your scores indicate room for improvement.

Scores of 6 to 8   Your health practices in this area are good, but there is room for improvement. Look again at the items you answered with a "Sometimes" or "Almost Never." What changes can you make to improve your score? Even a small change can often help you achieve better health.

Scores of 3 to 5   Your health risks are showing! Would you like more information about the risks you are facing and about why it is important for you to change these behaviors? Perhaps you need help in deciding how to successfully make the changes you desire. In either case, help is available.

Scores of 0 to 2   Obviously, you were concerned enough about your health to take the test, but your answers show that you may be taking serious and unnecessary risks with your health. Perhaps you are not aware of the risks and what to do about them. You can easily get the information and help you need to improve, if you wish. The next step is up to you.

YOU Can Start Right Now!

In the test you just completed were numerous suggestions to help you reduce your risk of disease and premature death. Here are some of the most significant:

Avoid cigarettes. Cigarette smoking is the single most important preventable cause of illness and early death. It is especially risky for pregnant women and their unborn babies. Persons who stop smoking reduce their risk of getting heart disease and cancer. So if you're a cigarette smoker, think twice about lighting that next cigarette. If you choose to continue smoking, try decreasing the number of cigarettes you smoke and switching to a low tar and nicotine brand.

Follow sensible drinking habits. Alcohol produces changes in mood and behavior. Most people who drink are able to control their intake of alcohol and to avoid undesired, and often harmful, effects. Heavy, regular use of alcohol can lead to cirrhosis of the liver, a leading cause of death. Also, statistics clearly show that mixing drinking and driving is often the cause of fatal or crippling accidents. So if you drink, do it wisely and in moderation. ***Use care in taking drugs.*** Today's greater use of drugs — both legal and illegal — is one of our most serious health risks. Even some drugs prescribed by your doctor can be dangerous if taken when drinking alcohol or before driving. Excessive or continued use of tranquilizers (or "pep pills") can cause physical and mental problems. Using or experimenting with illicit drugs such as marijuana, heroin, cocaine, and PCP may lead to a number of damaging effects or even death.

Eat sensibly. Overweight individuals are at greater risk for diabetes, gall bladder disease, and high blood pressure. So it makes good sense to maintain proper weight. But good eating habits also mean holding down the amount of fat (especially saturated fat), cholesterol, sugar and salt in your diet. If you must snack, try nibbling on fresh fruits and vegetables. You'll feel better — and look better, too.

Exercise regularly. Almost everyone can benefit from exercise — and there's some form of exercise almost everyone can do. (If you have any doubt, check first with your doctor.) Usually, as little as 20–30 minutes of vigorous exercise three times a week will help you have a healthier heart, eliminate excess weight, tone up sagging muscles, and sleep better. Think how much difference all these improvements could make in the way you feel!

Learn to handle stress. Stress is a normal part of living; everyone faces it to some degree. The causes of stress can be good or bad, desirable or undesirable (such as a promotion on the job or the loss of a spouse). Properly handled, stress need not be a problem. But unhealthy responses to stress — such as driving too fast or erratically, drinking too much, or prolonged anger or grief — can cause a variety of physical and mental problems. Even on a very busy day, find a few minutes to slow down and relax. Talking over a problem with someone you trust can often help you find a satisfactory solution. Learn to distinguish between things that are "worth fighting about" and things less important.

Be safety conscious. Think "safety first" at home, at work, at school, at play, and on the highway. Buckle seat belts and obey traffic rules. Keep poisons and weapons out of the reach of children, and keep emergency numbers by your telephone. When the unexpected happens, you'll be prepared.

Where Do You Go From Here:

Start by asking yourself a few frank questions: *Am I really doing all I can to be as healthy as possible? What steps can I take to feel better? Am I willing to begin now?* If you scored low in one or more *sections* of the test, decide what changes you want to make for improvement. You might pick that aspect of your lifestyle where you feel you have the best chance for success and tackle that one first. Once you have improved your score there, go on to other areas.

If you already have tried to change your health habits (to stop smoking or exercise regularly, for example), don't be discouraged if you haven't yet succeeded. The difficulty you have encountered may be due to influences you've never really thought about — such as advertising — or to a lack of support and encouragement. Understanding these influences is an important step toward changing the way they affect you.

There's Help Available. In addition to personal actions you can take on your own, there are community programs and groups (such as the YMCA or the local chapter of the American Heart Association) that can assist you and your family to make the changes you want to make. If you want to know more about these groups or about health risks, contact your local health department or the National Health Information Clearinghouse. There's a lot you can do to stay healthy or to improve your health — and there are organizations that can help you. Start a new HEALTH-STYLE today!

Select Bibliography

American College of Sports Medicine. *Guidelines for Exercise Testing and Prescription*. Baltimore: Williams & Wilkins, 1995.

American Cancer Society. *Cancer Book*. New York: ACS, 1986.

American College of Sports Medicine. "The Recommended Quantity and Quality of Exercise for Developing and Maintaining Cardiorespiratory and Muscular Fitness in Healthy Adults." *Medicine and Science in Sports and Exercise*, 22: (1990), 265–274.

Bennett, E. G., and D. Woolf (Editors). *Substance Abuse*. Albany, NY: Delmar Publishers, 1991.

Brownell, K., and J. P. Forey. *Handbook of Eating Disorders*. New York: Basic Books, 1986.

Byrne, K. *Understanding and Managing Cholesterol: A Guide for Wellness Professional*. Champaign, IL: Human Kinetics Books, 1991.

Coleman, E. *Eating for Endurance*. Palo Alto, CA: Bull Publishing, 1992.

Cristian, J. L., and J. L. Greger. *Nutrition for Living*. Menlo Park, CA: Benjamin/Cummings Publishing, 1991.

Fox, E. L., R. W. Bowers, and M. L. Fossand. *The Physiological Basis for Exercise and Sport*. Philadelphia: Saunders College Publishing, 1993.

Girdano, D., and G. Everly. *Controlling Stress and Tension: A Holistic Approach*. Englewood Cliffs, NJ: Prentice Hall, 1990.

Hafen, B. Q., and W. W. K. Hoeger. *Wellness: Guidelines for a Healthy Lifestyle*. Englewood, CO: Morton Publishing, 1994.

Hesson, J. L. *Weight Training for Life*. Englewood, CO: Morton Publishing, 1995.

Heyward, V. H. *Advanced Fitness Assessment & Exercise Prescription*. Champaign, IL: Human Kinetics, 1991.

Hoeger, W. W. K. *Lifetime Physical Fitness and Wellness: A Personalized Program*. Englewood, CO: Morton Publishing, 1995.

Hoeger, W. W. K., and S. A. Hoeger. *Principles and Labs for Physical Fitness and Wellness*. Englewood, CO: Morton Publishing, 1994.

Johnson, E. M. *What You Can Do to Avoid AIDS*. New York: Random House, 1992.

Kirschmann, J. D. *Nutrition Almanac.* New York: McGraw-Hill Book, 1989.

McArdle, W. D., F. I. Katch, and V. L. Katch. *Essentials of Exercise Physiology.* Philadelphia: Lea & Febiger, 1994.

National Academy of Sciences: Institute of Medicine. *Eat for Life: the Food and Nutrition Board's Guide to Reducing Your Risk of Chronic Disease* edited by C. E. Woteki and P. R. Thomas. Washington, DC: National Academy Press, 1992.

Pfeiffer, R. P, and B. C. Mangus. *Concepts of Athletic Training.* Boston: Jones and Bartlett Publishers, 1995.

Schafer, W. *Stress Management for Wellness.* Ft. Worth, TX: HBJ College Publishers, 1992.

Selye, H. *The Stress of Life.* New York: McGraw-Hill Book, 1978.

Whitney, E. N., and S. R. Rolfes. *Understanding Nutrition.* St. Paul, MN: West Publishing, 1993.

Wilmore, J. H., and D. L. Costill. *Training for Sport and Activity.* Dubuque, IA: Wm. C. Brown Publishers, 1988.

Glossary

Acquired immunodeficiency syndrome (AIDS) Final stage of infection by human immunodeficiency virus (HIV), which destroys the immune system.

Addiction Compulsive and uncontrollable behavior(s) or use of substance(s), most frequently drugs.

Adipose tissue Fat cells.

Aerobic dance *See* **Aerobics.**

Aerobic exercise Continuous exercise that involves major muscle groups and requires oxygen to produce the necessary energy to carry out the activity.

Aerobic fitness *See* **Cardiorespiratory endurance.**

Aerobics A series of exercise routines performed to music.

Agility The ability to quickly and efficiently change body position and direction.

AIDS *See* **Acquired immunodeficiency syndrome.**

Altruism True concern for and action on behalf of others

Amenorrhea Cessation of regular menstrual flow.

Amino acids Chemical compounds that contain nitrogen, carbon, hydrogen, and oxygen; the basic building blocks the body uses to form different types of protein.

Anabolic steroids Synthetic versions of the male sex hormone testosterone, which promotes muscle development and hypertrophy.

Anaerobic exercise Exercise that does not require oxygen to produce the necessary energy to carry out the activity.

Angiogenesis Capillary (blood vessel) formation into cancerous tumors.

Anorexia nervosa An eating disorder characterized by self-imposed starvation to lose and maintain very low body weight.

Antioxidants Compounds such as the vitamins C, E, beta-carotene, and the mineral selenium, which prevent oxygen from combining with other substances so that it may cause damage; thought to play a key role in preventing heart disease and cancer.

Atherosclerosis Cardiovascular disease characterized by plaque formation or buildup of fatty tissue in inner layers of artery walls.

Balance The ability to maintain the body in proper equilibrium.

Ballistic (dynamic) stretching Flexibility exercises performed using jerky, rapid, and bouncy movements.

Basal metabolic rate (BMR) The lowest level of oxygen consumption (uptake) necessary to sustain life.

Behavior modification A process to change destructive or negative behaviors permanently for positive behaviors that will lead to better health and well-being.

Benign Noncancerous.

Beta-carotene A precursor to vitamin A; an antioxidant which plays a role in disease prevention.

Biomechanics Science that studies the motion of humans and the effects that forces have on the body.

Blood lipids Fat-soluble substances in the body.

Blood pressure The force of blood exerted against artery walls.

Body composition Fat and nonfat components of the human body.

Breathing techniques Stress management method in which the individual concentrates on "breathing away" the tension and inhaling fresh air to the entire body.

Bulimia An eating disorder characterized by a pattern of binge eating and purging to attempt to lose and maintain low body weight.

Calorie A unit to measure energy value of food and physical activity; the amount of heat necessary to raise the temperature of 1 gram of water 1 degree Centigrade; short term for kilocalorie.

Cancer Group of diseases characterized by uncontrolled growth and spread of abnormal cells into malignant tumors.

Carbohydrates Compounds containing carbon, hydrogen, and oxygen; major source of energy for the human body.

Carcinogens Substances that contribute to formation of cancers.

Carcinoma in situ Encapsulated tumor that is found at an early stage and has not spread.

Cardiorespiratory endurance Ability of lungs, heart, and blood vessels to deliver adequate amounts of oxygen to the cells to meet the demands of prolonged (aerobic) physical activity.

Cardiorespiratory fitness *See* **Cardiorespiratory endurance**.

Cardiorespiratory training zone Recommended exercise heart rate range to cause development of cardiorespiratory endurance.

Cardiovascular diseases Degenerative conditions that involve the heart and the circulatory system (blood vessels).

Cellulite Term frequently used in reference to lumpy fat deposits; actually enlarged fat cells resulting from excessive accumulation of body fat.

CHD *See* **Coronary heart disease**.

Cholesterol A waxy substance that is technically a steroid alcohol found only in animal fats and oil.

Chronic diseases Illnesses that develop over a long time, usually associated with unhealthy lifestyle factors (e.g., hypertension, atherosclerosis, coronary disease, strokes, diabetes, and cancer).

Chronic obstructive pulmonary disease (COPD) Any of the several diseases that limit air flow, such as chronic bronchitis and emphysema.

Chronological age Actual, numerical age of the individual.

Concentric contraction Shortening of fibers during muscle contraction.

Cool-down Last segment of exercise session, spent in gradually decreasing the intensity of exercise.

Coordination The integration of the nervous and the muscular systems to produce correct, graceful, and harmonious body movements.

Coronary heart disease (CHD) Condition caused by obstruction of coronary arteries by plaque formation.

Criterion referenced standard *See* **Health-fitness standard.**

Cross-training Combining two or more fitness activities.

Cruciferous vegetables Plants that produce cross-shaped leaves (cauliflower, broccoli, cabbage, Brussels sprouts, and kohlrabi); seem to have a protective effect against cancer.

Daily values (DVs) Government food labeling that includes the percentage of recommended daily amounts of nutrients.

Dehydration Loss of body water below normal volume.

Deoxyribonucleic acid (DNA) Genetic material, substance of which genes are made.

Diabetes mellitus Condition wherein blood glucose is unable to enter the cells because the pancreas either totally stops producing insulin or produces an insufficient amount for the body's needs.

Dietary fiber Material in plant foods that the human body cannot digest; a carbohydrate.

DNA *See* **Deoxyribonucleic acid.**

Duration of exercise Length of time of each exercise bout.

Dynamic stretching *See* **Ballistic stretching**

Dysmenorrhea Painful menstruation.

Eccentric contraction Lengthening of fibers during muscle contraction.

ECG *See* **Electrocardiogram**.

EKG *See* **Electrocardiogram**.

Electrocardiogram (ECG or EKG) A recording of the electrical activity of the heart.

Endurance *See* **Cardiorespiratory endurance**; **Muscular endurance**.

Energy balancing equation States that when caloric intake equals caloric output, weight remains unchanged.

Epidemiology Science that studies the relationship between diverse factors (lifestyle and environmental) and occurrence of disease.

Essential fat Minimal amount of body fat needed for normal physiological functions; about 3% of total fat in men and 12% in women.

Exercise ECG An exercise test during which the workload is increased gradually (until the subject reaches maximal fatigue) with electrocardiographic monitoring throughout the test.

Exercise intolerance Physical aversion to exercise conducted at intensity levels beyond a person's functional capacity.

Exercise tolerance test *See* **Exercise electrocardiogram**.

Fats Compounds made by a combination of triglycerides; a source of energy to the body.

Fiber *See* **Dietary Fiber**.

Fight-or-flight mechanism Physiological response of the body to stress, which prepares the individual to take action by stimulating the vital defense systems.

Flexibility The ability of a joint to move freely through its full range of motion.

Free fatty acids (FFA) *See* **Triglycerides**.

Free radicals *See* **Oxygen free radicals**.

Frequency of exercise Number of training sessions per week.

Functional age Physiological age of the individual; usually lower than chronological (actual) age in fit people and vice versa in unfit people.

HDL *See* **High density lipoprotein**.

Health-fitness (criterion referenced) standards Minimum fitness standards to decrease risk of disease significantly.

Health-related fitness Refers to fitness components that, when enhanced, lead to better health (cardiorespiratory endurance, body composition, muscular strength and endurance, and muscular flexibility).

Heart rate reserve The difference between the maximal heart rate and the resting heart rate.

Heat cramps Muscle cramps caused by heat-induced changes in electrolyte balance in muscle cells.

Heat exhaustion Heat-related condition; symptoms include fainting, dizziness, profuse sweating, cold clammy skin, headaches, and a rapid, weak pulse.

Heat stroke Heat-related emergency; symptoms include serious disorientation, warm dry skin, no sweating, rapid pulse, vomiting, diarrhea, unconsciousness, and high body temperature.

Hemoglobin Substance in blood that carries oxygen from lungs to all body tissues.

High-density lipoprotein (HDL) Cholesterol-transporting molecules in the blood (the "good" cholesterol); offers protection against some forms of cardiovascular disease.

High-impact aerobics (HIA) Actions in which both feet leave the floor at the same time momentarily.

High physical-fitness standards Required criteria to achieve a high level of fitness; level of moderate to vigorous activity without causing undue fatigue.

HIV *See* **Human Immunodeficiency Virus.**

Human immunodeficiency virus (HIV) Virus that causes acquired immunodeficiency syndrome (AIDS).

Hypertension Chronically elevated blood pressure; blood pressures above 140/90, according to the American Heart Association.

Hypertrophy *See* **Muscle hypertrophy**.

Hypokinetic diseases Illnesses associated with a lack of physical activity (e.g., hypertension, coronary heart disease, obesity, and diabetes).

Intensity of exercise How hard a person has to exercise to improve cardiorespiratory endurance.

Isokinetic training Strength-training method in which the speed of the muscle contraction is kept constant because the equipment (machine) provides an accommodating resistance to match the user's force through the range of motion.

Isometric training Strength-training method that involves a muscle contraction producing little or no movement, such as pushing or pulling against immovable objects.

Isotonic training Strength-training method that involves a muscle contraction with movement, such as lifting an object over the head.

Kilocalorie The amount of heat necessary to raise the temperature of 1 kilogram of water 1 degree Centigrade; usually shortened to "calorie."

LDL *See* **Low density lipoprotein.**

Lean body mass Body weight without body fat.

Locus of control The extent to which a person believes he or she can influence the external environment.

Low-density lipoprotein (LDL) Cholesterol-transporting molecules in the blood (the "bad" cholesterol) that increases the risk of some forms of cardiovascular disease.

Low-impact aerobics (LIA) Exercise in which at least one foot is in contact with the floor at all times.

Macronutrients Nutrients that the body requires in proportionately large amounts daily.

Malignant Cancerous.

Malignant melanoma Deadliest of all types of skin cancer. Tumors grow at a rapid rate and readily spread to other parts of the body if not treated at an early stage.

Maximal oxygen uptake (VO$_{2max}$) The maximum amount of oxygen that the body is able to utilize per minute of physical activity, commonly expressed in ml/kg/min.

Melanoma A malignant skin cancer.

Metabolism All energy and material transformations that occur within living cells necessary to sustain life.

Metastasis The movement of bacteria or body cells from one part of the body to the other; usually in reference to cancer.

MET (metabolic equivalent) A measurement unit of resting energy expenditure; 1 MET is the equivalent of 3.5 ml/kg/min.

Micronutrients Vitamins and minerals that the body requires in small amounts.

Minerals Inorganic elements found in the body and in food, essential for normal body functions.

Mode of exercise Type of exercise with the respect to effect or outcome.

Motivation The desire and will to do something.

Muscle hypertrophy Muscle's ability to increase in size.

Muscular endurance (localized muscular endurance) The ability of a muscle to exert submaximal force repeatedly over a period of time (for example, 30 repetitions on a bench-press exercise); usually implies a specific muscle group (e.g., chest, thighs, abdominals).

Muscular flexibility *See* **Flexibility**.

Muscular strength The ability of a muscle to exert maximum force against resistance (for example, 1 repetition maximum [1 RM] on the bench press exercise).

Nonmelanoma skin cancer Cancer that grows directly from the original site but does not metastasize to other regions of the body.

Nutrient Substance found in food that provide energy, regulate metabolism, and help with growth and repair of body tissues.

Nutrient density Ratio of nutrients to calories in food.

Nutrition Science that studies the relationship of foods to optimal health and performance.

Obesity An excessive accumulation of body fat, about 30% above recommended body weight according to body size.

Oligomenorrhea Irregular menstrual cycles.

One repetition maximum (1 RM) The maximal amount of resistance (weight) an individual is able to lift in a single effort.

Osteoporosis Softening, deterioration, or loss of total body bone.

Overload principle Training concept stating that the demands placed on a system (cardiorespiratory, muscular) must be increased systematically and progressively over a period of time to cause physiologic adaptation (development or improvement).

Overweight Excess weight when compared to a given standard.

Oxygen free radicals Substances formed during metabolism that attack and damage proteins and lipids, in particular the cell membrane and DNA, leading to development of diseases such as heart disease, cancer, and emphysema.

Percent body fat Total amount of fat in the body based on person's weight; includes both essential and storage fat.

Physical fitness The general capacity to adapt and respond favorably to physical effort, capable of meeting the ordinary as well as the unusual demands of daily life safely and effectively without being overly fatigued and still have energy left for leisure and recreational activities.

Phytochemicals Food substances that help prevent disease, especially cancer.

Plyometrics Exercise that requires forceful jumps or springing off the ground immediately after landing from a previous jump.

PNF *See* **Proprioceptive neuromuscular facilitation**.

Power The ability to produce maximum force in the shortest time.

Progressive muscle relaxation Stress management technique involving contraction and relaxation of muscle groups throughout the body.

Proprioceptive neuromuscular facilitation (PNF) Stretching technique in which muscles are stretched out progressively with intermittent isometric contractions.

Proteins Complex organic compounds containing nitrogen and formed by combinations of amino acids; the main substances used in the body to build and repair tissues such as muscles, blood, internal organs, skin, hair, nails, and bones; also part of hormones, antibodies, and enzymes.

RDA *See* **Recommended dietary allowances**.

Reaction time The time required to initiate a response to a given stimulus.

Recommended dietary allowances (RDAs) Daily recommended intakes of nutrients for normal, healthy people in the United States.

Repetition The number of times a given action is performed (for example, 12 repetitions on the bench press exercise).

Resistance (in strength training) Amount of weight lifted.

Resting metabolic rate Amount of energy (expressed in milliliters of oxygen per minute or total calories per day) required during nonactive conditions to sustain proper body function.

Risk factors Lifestyle and genetic components that may lead to disease.

Set (in strength training) Number of repetitions (e. g., one set of 12 repetitions) per exercise.

Setpoint Weight control theory that indicates that each body has an established weight and strongly attempts to maintain that weight.

Sexually transmitted diseases (STDs) Diseases spread through sexual contact.

Shin splint Injury to the lower leg characterized by pain and irritation at the front of the leg.

Side stitch Sharp pain in the side during exercise.

Skill-related fitness Refers to fitness components beyond health-related fitness that enhance athletic performance (agility, balance, coordination, reaction time, power, and speed).

Skinfold thickness Technique to assess body composition, including percent body fat, by measuring the thickness of a double fold of skin at different body sites.

Slow-sustained (static) stretching (flexibility) Technique in which the muscles are lengthened gradually through a joint's complete range of motion and the final position is held for a few seconds.

Specificity of training Principle stating that exercise programs must be aimed at the desired outcome.

Speed The ability to rapidly propel the body or a part of the body from one point to another.

Spirituality An affirmation of life in a relationship with God, self, community, and environment that nurtures and celebrates wholeness.

Spot reducing Fallacious theory that claims that exercising a specific body part will result in significant fat reduction in that area.

Static stretching *See* **Slow-sustained stretching**.

STDs *See* **Sexually transmitted diseases**.

Step aerobics A relatively new form of aerobics using a combination of stepping and arm movements and benches.

Storage fat Body fat in excess of the essential fat; stored in adipose tissue.

Strength *See* **Muscular strength**.

Stress Nonspecific response of the human organism to any demand placed upon it.

Stress test *See* **Exercise ECG**.

Tolerable weight A standard that is not quite "ideal" but is "acceptable."

Triglycerides Fats formed by combination of glycerol and three fatty acids.

Very low density lipoprotein (VLDL) Triglyceride-, cholesterol-, and phospholipid-transporting molecules in the blood.

Vitamins Organic substances essential for normal metabolism, growth, and development of the body.

VLDL *See* **Very low density lipoprotein**.

VO$_{2max}$ *See* **Maximal oxygen uptake**

Waist-to-hip ratio Test designed by a panel of scientists appointed by National Academy of Sciences and Dietary Guidelines Advisory Council for U. S. Departments of Agriculture and Health and Human Services to assess potential risk for diseases associated with obesity.

Warm-up The first segment of an exercise consisting of general calisthenics or stretching exercises.

Water The most important nutrient, involved in almost every vital bodily process.

Wellness The constant and deliberate effort to stay healthy and achieve the highest potential for well-being; implies adoption of healthy lifestyle factors that will decrease the risk for disease and enhance well-being.

Index

Cardiovascular disease
  and antioxidants, 99
  and death rates, 3, 9, 122, 123
  incidence of, 4, 123
  and nutrition , 88, 90
  risk factors for, 5, 114, 123, 124,
    126, 146-147
  and smoking, 129
Cellulite, 114
Centers for Disease Control and
    Prevention, 143
CHD. *See* Cardiovascular disease
Chemical dependency, 141-142
Childbearing, 9
Chlamydia, 142
Cholesterol, 88, 89, 126, 129
Chronic conditions
  incidence of, 4
  nutrition and, 88
  related to lack of physical activity, 3
  risks for, 9, 20
Chronic and obstructive pulmonary
    disease (COPD), 3, 122, 139
Cigarettes. *See* Tobacco use
Clothing, 149, 153, 154, 155
  when cycling, 76
  during pregnancy, 158
Cocaine, 149-150
Coffee, 161
Commitment, 118, 168
Confidence, 13
Cool-down, 29, 48, 84
Cooper, Kenneth, 4, 71, 101
Coordination, 7 81, 83
Cross-country skiing, 78-79
Cross-training, 70, 77-78
Cycling, 58-59, 75-76, 114

Daily Values (DV), 92
Death. *See also* Mortality rate
  leading causes of, 3
Dehydration, 154, 161
Depression , 9
Diabetes, 9, 88, 124, 125, 128, 146
Diet
  anti-cancer, 136
  for athletes, 161-162
  balanced, 90-92, 93, 101, 122
  industry, 109
  and LDL-lowering guidelines, 127,
    128
  low-calorie, 111
  low-fat, 160
  supplementation, 96, 99-101
  typical, 87-88
DNA, 135, 136
Duration of exercise, 46, 48
Dynamic strength. *See* Isotonic
Dysmenorrhea, 157

Eating, healthy, 118-119. *See also*
  Diet; Nutrition

Eating disorders, 33, 101-103
Electrocardiograms, 22, 114, 124, 128,
    129
Endurance, 7
  cardiorespiratory, 6-7, 20, 21-22,
    25, 42, 71, 74, 81, 124, 125, 148
  muscular, 7, 25-26, 48-49, 51
Energy, 22, 25, 87, 88, 89, 109, 114
Energy-balancing equation, 109, 112
Environment
  and cancer, 136, 139
  and free radicals, 99
  and health, 4, 122
  temperature of, 153, 154, 155
Equipment, exercise, 165
Estrogen, 138-139, 158
Evaluation, 15-16. *See also* Assessment
Exercise
  Aero-belt, 76-77
  aerobic, 21, 46, 58, 59-60, 72, 113,
    145-146, 154
  and aging, 162
  and blood donation, 147
  compulsive, 132
  and diabetes, 128
  duration, 46, 48
  equipment, 166
  frequency, 48, 52, 55
  intensity, 43, 45-46, 55, 81, 85,
    149, 150
  intolerance, 148
  mode, 46, 49, 50
  during pregnancy, 157-158
  readiness for, 42
  and stress, 130, 132
  time of day for, 149-150
  vigorous, 10, 20, 43
  warm-up, 22
  and weight management, 111, 112-
    113, 118

Facilities, health-fitness, 165-166
Fat
  body, 4, 33, 34, 111, 112, 114, 115,
    124, 125, 127, 146, 155
  dietary, 14, 87, 88-89, 90-92, 93,
    101, 127, 136
Fatigue, 9, 51, 61
  chronic, 132
Females
  and anorexia nervosa, 101
  and essential fat, 33
  and flexibility, 29
  and heart disease, 123, 134-135
  and iron, 159
  and osteoporosis, 158
  physiological differences from males,
    155-156
  pregnant, 153
  and skinfold sites, 34
  and wasit-to-hip ratio, 39

Fiber, dietary, 87, 88, 93, 127, 128,
    136
Fight or flight, 130
Fitness, 167
  benefits of, 8
  cardiorespiratory, 21, 46
  definition of, 6
  health-related, 6-7, 19, 20, 25, 46,
    48, 81, 83, 109
  in older people, 25, 162
  skill-related, 6, 7-8, 81, 83, 84
  standards, 20
  of youth, 4
Fixx, Jim, 71
Flexibility, muscular, 9, 28-29, 53-54,
    56, 83, 148
  and aging, 29
  assessing, 29-33
  exercises for, 54-55, 74
  differences in men and women, 29
Fluid replacement, 154, 160-161
Folacin, 100
Food and Drug Administration, 92
Food Guide Pyramid, 93, 94-95
Food label, 92
Force. *See* Strength
Framingham Heart Study, 126
Fraud, 164-165
Free radicals. *See* Antioxidants
Free weights, 50
Frequency of exercise, 48, 52, 55
Frostbite, 154, 155
Fruits, 93, 99, 136

Genetic factors
  in anorexia nervosa, 101
  in body type, 156
  in cancer, 135
  in COPD, 139
  in diabetes, 128
  in disease, 4, 122
  in fitness, 83, 84
  and flexibility, 28
  in weight, 108, 110
Genital warts, 142
Goals, 13
  setting, 14, 15-16, 61-62, 118

Gonorrhea, 142

HDL cholesterol, 89, 124, 125, 126-
    127, 128, 129
Health care, 4
  costs of, 6
Health fitness standards, 20, 46, 48,
    109
Healthy People 2000, 10-11, 12
Heart disease, 9, 88. *See also* Cardio-
    vascular disease
  and age, 134
  and stress, 130

Heart rate, 46, 85
  in cycling, 75
  exercise, 72, 85
  maximal, 45, 73, 75
  recovery, 148
  reserve, 45
  resting, 45
  and smoking, 129
  in water aerobics, 74
Heat
  cramps, 153
  exhaustion, 153
  stroke, 153-154
Height/weight charts, 33-34
Heredity. See Genetic factors
Herpes, 142
Hesson, James, 156
High-impact aerobics (HIA). See
  Aerobics
Hiking, 70
HIV, 142-143
Hormone replacement therapy, 158
Hypertension. See Blood pressure
Hypertrophy, muscle, 25, 51, 155,
  156, 163
Hypokinetic diseases, 3
Hypothermia, 154-155

Immune system, 135, 140, 142
Injuries, 58, 150
  in aerobics, 59
  in cross-training, 77
  when cycling, 75-76
  from HIA, 72
  in in-line skating, 79
  in jogging/running, 58, 71
  knee, 59-60
  preventing, 20, 29, 55, 83, 86
  risk for, 51, 54, 61, 114
  in step aerobics, 72
  in stair climbing, 80
  in water aerobics, 74
Intensity of exercise, 43, 45-46, 55,
  81, 149, 150
  in aerobics, 72-73
  when cycling, 75
  for in-line skating, 79
  during pregnancy, 157
  in stair climbing, 80
  in water, 73, 75
International Dance Exercise
  Association (IDEA), 166
Interval training, 77
Iron deficiency, 96, 158-159
Isokinetc equipment, 50
Isometric contractions, 49-50, 54, 55
Isotonic
  strength, 49-50
  training, 50

Jogging/running, 58, 71

Junk food, 88

LDL cholesterol, 89, 124, 126, 127,
  146
Lean body mass, 33, 34, 39-40, 111,
  113, 114
LIA. See Aerobics
Lifestyle
  healthy, 4, 5, 8, 163. See also Well-
    ness
  negative, 3, 121, 122, 124, 135, 147
  sedentary, 10, 29, 53, 122
Lipids, 125, 126, 147. See also Fat
Lipoproteins, 126
Locus of control, l1, 13
Longevity, 9, 10, 81, 140
L-impact aerobics (LIA). See Aerobics

Macronutrients, 88
Males
  and essential fat, 33
  and flexibility, 29
  and heart disease, 123, 134-135
  physiological differences from
    females, 155-156
  and skinfold sites, 34
  and waist-to-hip ratio, 39
Marijuana, 141
Maximal heart rate (MHR), 45, 73,
  129
Metabolism, 96, 136
  and diet, 111, 114, 117
  resting, 25, 111
METs, 81
MIA. See Aerobics
Micronutrients, 88
Minerals, 90, 100
Mode of exercise
  in cardiorespiratory training, 46
  in flexibility training, 53-54
  in strength training, 49-51
Moderate-impact aerobics (MIA). See
  Aerobics
Monitoring, 14-15
Mortality rate, 9, 10, 33, 108, 122,
  134-135, 140
  and lifestyle, 121
  and tobacco use, 138
Motivation, 9, 11, 16, 61, 118
  lack of, 13, 14
Muscular
  cramps, 152-153
  endurance, 7, 25, 26, 48-49, 51
  flexibility, 9, 28-29, 53-55
  hypertrophy, 25, 155, 156, 163
  soreness and stiffness, 150-152
  strength, 7, 25-27, 48-49

National Academy of Sciences, 39, 92
National Cholesterol Education Program (NCEP), 126, 127

National Health Information Clearinghouse, 122
National Interfaith Coalition on Aging,
  139
Nutrients, 87
  analysis, 93, 96, 115
  essential, 88-90
  supplementation, 96

Obesity, 33, 34, 35, 107, 108, 111
  and cancer, 108, 136, 138
  and diabetes, 128
  and heart disease, 126
  and nutrition, 88
  and water aerobics, 74
Oligomenorrhea, 158
1.0-Mile Walk Test, 24-25
1.5-Mile Run Test, 22
1 RM, 26, 51
Osteoporosis, 88, 158
Overload
  muscle, 43, 50
  principle, 49, 53
Overtraining, 52, 100, 132
Overweight, 34, 83, 108, 114. See
  also Obesity
  and deep-water running, 71
  and diabetes, 128
  and low-back pain, 56
  numbers of, 107
  and swimming, 73
  and water aerobics, 74
Oxygen, 96
  uptake, 21, 22, 45, 74, 155, 163

Paffenbarger, Ralph, 9, 147
Pain, 55, 86
Passive smoke. See Secondhand smoke
Peer support, 14
Percent body fat, 33, 34, 35, 109, 110,
  114
Perspiration, 160-161
Physical fitness. See Fitness
Physical inactivity, 124-125
Phytochemicals, 93, 136, 138
Plastic elongation , 54
Plyometrics, 72-73
Pollution. See Environment
Posture, 9, 29, 56
  in step aerobics, 60
  while walking, 58
Power, 7, 81, 83
Pregnancy, exercise during, 157-158
President's Council on Physical Fitness
  and Sports, 48
Prevention
  of accidents/injury, 139, 145
  of cancer, 136, 139
  of heart disease, 124, 126, 146
  of illness, 4, 7, 11, 20, 48, 93, 122,
    135